Endangered Private Practice

Endangered Private Practice

Surviving Health Care Reform

Ronald R. Hixson

JASON ARONSON
Lanham • Boulder • New York • Toronto • Plymouth, UK

Published by Jason Aronson
A wholly owned subsidiary of The Rowman & Littlefield Publishing Group, Inc.
4501 Forbes Boulevard, Suite 200, Lanham, Maryland 20706
www.rowman.com

10 Thornbury Road, Plymouth PL6 7PP, United Kingdom

British Library Cataloguing in Publication Information Available

Library of Congress Cataloging-in-Publication Data

Hixson, Ronald, author.
Endangered private practice : surviving health care reform / Ronald R. Hixson.
p. cm.
Includes bibliographical references.
ISBN 978-0-7657-0935-6 (cloth : alk. paper) -- ISBN 978-0-7657-0936-3 (electronic)
I. Title. [DNLM: 1. Private Practice--United States. 2. Health Care Reform--United States. 3. Health Services--United States. 4. Practice Management, Medical--economics--United States. WB 50 AA1]
RA971
362.1068--dc23

2013029106

The paper used in this publication meets the minimum requirements of American National Standard for Information Sciences Permanence of Paper for Printed Library Materials, ANSI/NISO Z39.48-1992.

Printed in the United States of America

This book is dedicated to the memory of my ancestors who contributed to my genetic pathways that has influenced my decisions of a career of service for the less fortunate and more vulnerable to political and economic strife:

My maternal pathway

Hugo Paul Dorn
&
Alice Mae Brown Dorn

***

And my paternal pathway

William Henry Hixson
&
Margaret Horst Hixson

Contents

Acknowledgements

This book is an accumulation of influences from Art Hauck, an educator and independent thinker who lived, wrote, and challenged young minds at Union College, Lincoln, Nebraska and where he shared his love of books. Raymond Potterf, MD, PhD is a psychiatrist who has been a mentor and a strong resource for understanding symptomology. Dr. Potterf taught me the value of framing the question when investigating symptoms and following their pathways from body to mind and back. Moises Rodriguez, MD psychiatrist has shared his keen insight into symptoms and treatment on many difficult and complex cases. Primary care physicians have been a source of professional guidance and support, and I have learned so much in their field with their willingness to explore difficult questions in the treatment of challenging cases. Others who have added critical comments after reading the manuscript include Herbert Garfield, MD, Hector Trevino, MD, Nicholas Cummings, PhD, ScD, Paul McCollum, PhD, Herbert Shriver, PhD, JD, Micheale Dunlap, PsyD, Jerry Diehl, PhD, John Thompson, PA-C, Michael Luna, RPh, Patricia Penilla, RN, Michael Krumper, LSW, Mark Harris, LSW, Dana Unruh, LPC, and J. Rodriguez, MA. For these and my many friends and colleagues who have both encouraged me as well as offered their own experiences, I remain in their debt.

To my editor, Cheryl Barnett, I am forever grateful for the care and passion you entered into this project with and never left it until it was done. Until one has had his or her work challenged and a better way of presenting a concept offered, it is hard to explain the bond that is shared for a project. Any success that comes from this book is due to Cheryl and her commitment to excellence.

To Amy King, Assistant Acquisitions Editor, and Kelly Blackburn, Assistant Editor, my sincere thanks for making the publication process transition smoothly from typed manuscript to published book.

Introduction

Dating back to the Civil War, health care shortages, application of treatment and services have been discussed, debated, and baby steps have been taken every decade or two and now have reached a pivotal time in history where health care has come of age and has left the mom-and-pop cottage industry that has been run over by the monster trucks of health maintenance organizations (HMOs). For those that have not noticed the gradual changes in the services, treatments, delivery processes, and administrative and financial services, the health care industry has shown a substantial growth over the past seven decades. The little steps are now behind us, and consumers, producers, and administrators are being pushed across the stage by the powerful winds of reform. Something is happening that the American Medical Association (AMA) fought hard against for the past 100 years: the loss of autonomy for their physicians and the loss of power to determine what procedure to use, which diagnosis is better, and where and when to refer a patient to a specialist or another physician for a second opinion.

> Reformers believed that competition among health plans would drive down costs as health plans, through primary care physicians (PCPs), managed the patient's care and bargained with providers (Enthovon, 1993, 2004, 2005). Health plans (HMOs, and preferred provider organizations (PPOs) were to negotiate aggressively with providers, monitor physicians to control waste, and limit the provision of unnecessary care. The original idea—that care would be managed *for the patient* by a management *of physicians* by health plan administrators intent on reducing costs, limiting services, and increasing margins (Porter and Teisberg, 2006, pp.76-77).

This notion marked the beginning of the foray into micromanagement of providers by corporations contracted with the government to cut costs of health care that suddenly received very lucrative contracts with states that was spawned by the Affordable Care Act (ACA), which was launched in 2010 under the guidance of President Obama. This new approach forges a closer relationship between the federal government, Wall Street corporations, other special interest groups, and state governments, the like of which has never been seen before. The stated goal of this legislation included making health care services (treatments and medications) accessible to all citizens. The ACT, as the ACA is now called, was implemented over four to five years due to all the new regulations on states, HMOs, and all those who function as providers including hospitals, clinics, and group practices. Wall Street is happy because the federal government has made a plan that addresses the administrative and financial weaknesses often pointed out as the villains ruining the health care industry. HMOs are thrilled, as it gives them a pot of gold to use in the administration of large Medicaid populations and the power of the federal and state legislature, judicial, and law enforcement agencies to accomplish their mission. States are thrilled because they have less to worry about administratively, and the HMOs are on the hook to make good on their agreement to promise to lower the Medicaid budget, which will then free up more revenue that the states can use to keep their state budgets balanced.

This book aims to contribute to this debate on health care reform but not from the economic or financial perspectives. Instead the focus is on explaining how and why private practice has become the scapegoat for managed care and to offer some options for those still in practice. During the health care industry's cottage period, private practice was created as a convenience similar to the mom-and-pop corner stores. Over the past three to four decades the health care industry has been expanding with increasing speed to meet the exploding demand for treatment and medications. Traditionally providers felt that they controlled their own destiny; however, today their time schedules, billing and collection processes, reimbursement rates, required licenses continuing educational requirements, and professional liability requirements have changed the one person office into a team of specialists, many of whom are not working in the office but are actually agents of an HMO or managed care organization (MCO) who now have more to say about the delivery of services then the provider does. When people suggest that the market is driving health care reform (Blouche, 2003), they are wrong; politicians are driving it for two reasons: to use its financial resources to pay down state and federal budgets and to control the providers who are producers in the marketplace. By controlling them you motivate them to leave the field or to do as required by state regulations. This amounts to *puppet health care*. When providers are controlled they will produce what the state asks, and not much more. The heart of practice is the producer who spends between $100,000 and $300,000, or even more, for their formal education. They then put their passion, combined with their education and experience, into years of financing and building their practice. Now some entity, without medical or mental health training and experience, is telling providers how to operate their practice or they will not receive any reimbursement, and will perhaps lose the contract with the HMO. This is the viewpoint of most veteran physicians and allied health providers as noted through personal conversations and in reading the literature provided.

The marketplace is a problem that the government cannot touch, the third rail, perhaps. The marketplace is where the patient is and where they determine their own needs. The owners of the HMOs are stockholders who demand a healthy dividend every quarter. Without such, the dividend clippers will be unhappy and may unload their stock. A corporation needs stockholders, and they are definitely in the business to make a profit. In the marketplace this is a natural expectation. Accusing producers of health care as criminals or to suggest that they are the reason for all the problems with the health care system is ludicrous. That's like blaming everyone on the professional football team for not reaching the Super Bowl. From the perspective of many health care producers, owners of the health care industry do not care what their position is, as long as the owners' investment pays dividends. Investors are the ones who own stocks in corporations that trade on Wall Street. This underlines how far apart the owners are from the health care producers who rely, for the most part, on their practice to make a profit so they can cash their payroll checks.

> According to the IRS, which recently released 2009 data from the 400 richest individual income tax returns, the real runaway growth in wealth has come from capital gains. In the last years of the bubble, the "Fortunate 400" made nearly half their income from capital gains (a.k.a.: profit from the rising value of an investment, such as stocks or property) and less than 10% of their income from old-fashioned wages.

> The average income of a top-400 earner grew by 650% between 1992 and 2007 to a whopping $344 million. Over that time, the average salary didn't even double. But the average capital gains haul increased by 1,200%. So how do the richest get richer? Not from their wages; from their investments (Thompson, 2012, p. 1).

Chapter One briefly discusses the history of the healthcare reform movement and addresses how the present structure is a threat to private practice and to the personal and professional autonomy, sense of integrity and ethics of the providers. The new structures coming out of the reform ACT of 2010 include structures that will be solicited and encouraged to do business as groups under the guidelines of the ACT.

Affordable care organizations (ACOs) include physicians and other health care providers who have the new technology to share confidential information among group members as part of the collaboration that the act supports for more quality care and less duplication of services. According to Bryant (2011) the Center of Medicaid and Medicare Services (CMS) began signing up approved ACOs in 2012. Other groups that are likely to be approved include Coordinating Care Organizations (CCOs), groups in network practice arrangements, hospitals employing multi-disciplinary professionals, providers in group practices such as a Professional Practice Association (PPAs), and Independent Practice Associations (IPAs). Any such group must have approval of CMS, which often works with the local state government to verify group credentials and to make sure they are compliant with the ACO requirements for IT, confidentiality, and quality control.

Chapter One introduces how providers are losing their practices and how they feel about it. Chapter Two discusses the major factors pushing the current winds of change and the power engine that drives the force of change. In Chapter Three we explore how providers of all healthcare disciplines are seldom ready to tackle the problems created by the business side of practice. In the past dozen years politics has had much more influence on the practice of healthcare. Chapter Four suggests ways to re-define one's niche in the marketplace given the changes presented in the previous chapters. Chapter Five focuses on creating value in a practice as a method of redemption for those who continue to carry a passion for one-on-one health care education and therapy. In Chapter Six we look into a crystal ball for future directions that healthcare reform may take, and then ask: Why isn't healthcare based on fundamental moral principals as much as on questions of healthcare quality? One cannot encourage the dialogue of healthcare treatments, finance, delivery, and quality without addressing one of the most dramatic articles of 2013: "The Bitter Pill", by Steven Brill.

This book will pick up where other books have shied away from such topics as risks and vulnerabilities of private practice. Hopefully such information will encourage action to protect the profession as well as the integrity of this profession even as we are pushed into group practice or professional networks (IPAs). This book ends with Brill's pill, but the author is keenly aware that we have not ended, but have only just begun to address the real costs of healthcare that begs for more; not in this book, but in books to come.

Chapter One

Turbulence Leads to Chaos

At a recent county medical association meeting in a south Texas rural community, several physicians were sharing concerns in regards to the rapid changes that seem to keep providers, as well as patients, off balance. One doctor asked, "How many of you are thinking of changing the way you practice?" Another physician responded that he was going to keep the patients he was currently seeing, but would not accept any more new patients with Medicaid and/or Medicare. Another physician solemnly shook his head and reported that he was thinking of closing his practice. Still another physician suggested that creating an Affordable Care Organization might offer an opportunity to continue in practice without continuing the flow of red ink. "Yes," answered one of his associates, "that could be an opportunity, but we would have to come up with a lot of capital to form one or to even join one. Then we would be expected to share in the cost of administration and management. More money would be sliding out the door before the first patient comes in." Similar conversations can be heard across state lines, as it is a general concern for all physicians, but it is not confined to primary care physicians because the reform movement affects every licensed health care provider.

Uncertainty and unexpected events can bring change, almost overnight, to any marketplace. Reform movements are created to change the political landscape, to challenge old concepts within different contexts that affect the way we practice our business. During the past decade the health care industry has had an extraordinary number of situations and events arise, including legislation that was not expected nor appreciated at the time. Like riding a roller coaster alone and blindfolded, one's senses are forced to try to regain balance and perception. This is the time to check the safety apparatus and to stymie the panic that is creeping up from the bowels. Providers are finding that they

1

have to worry more about the mechanics of practice than the quality of services. In the meantime the new HMO who administers their Medicaid claims is switching patients to other primary care physicians, reports a primary care physician, (PCP). He took out an advertisement in the local paper explaining to the public that patients have the right to stay with their PCP, but they may have to call the new HMO and start the paperwork to switch back. No wonder there is a mistrust of government, politicians, and corporate health care, which may explain why millions do not vote during any given election (Rago, 2011; Allen, 2010; Fraser, 2010; Thomma, 2009).

WHAT HAPPENED TO THE HEALTH CARE INDUSTRY?

Beginning with the early midwives, shamans, nurses, and doctors on horseback who would go out to farms to see patients, to the drastic shortages of medical and nursing care providers during the Civil War years, the early efforts to provide medical treatments for the sick and wounded was minimal. As more physicians and nurses became available, the health care field grew into a cottage industry that flourished during the war years of the 20th century. With the help of the GI Bill, returning veterans traded in their helmets and uniforms for the new uniforms of the medical and nursing professions. With the advent of X-rays came new physicians specializing in advanced technology and psychiatrists using new psychotropic medications. As more specialists entered the picture in the fields of internal medicine, orthopedics, pediatrics, neurology, and obstetrics expanded services, costs began to rise.

The many deaths and injuries during the Civil War seemed to bring to the public's attention the need for nurses and doctors with extensive knowledge and experience. When WWI began, the number of dead and wounded was even worse. It was during this time in our history that society seemed to wake up and discover the usefulness of insurance policies and the value of hospitals and health care providers. The first insurance policies written were fire and accident policies purchased during the Civil War days.

The first group policy giving comprehensive benefits was offered by Massachusetts Health Insurance of Boston in 1847. Insurance companies issued the first individual disability and illness policies in about 1890. In 1929, the first modern group health insurance plan was formed. A group of teachers in Dallas, Texas, contracted with Baylor Hospital for room, board, and medical services in exchange for a monthly fee. Several large life insurance companies entered the health insurance field in the 1930's and 1940's as the popularity of health insurance increased. In 1932 nonprofit organizations called Blue Cross or Blue Shield first offered group health plans. Blue Cross and Blue Shield Plans were successful because they involved discounted contracts negotiated with doctors and hospitals. In return for promises of increased volume and prompt payment, providers gave discounts to the Blue Cross and Shield plans (Neurosurgical.com, 2012).

During the next 25 years there was a slow growth of insurance companies selling policies to employers for their employees and competing with each other for providers and customers. Metropolitan and Prudential were two of the largest competitors to Blue Cross Blue Shield. In the late 1930s and early 1940s, Kaiser Permanente was established to serve the needs of thousands of Kaiser's employees in their steel, shipyards, and construction jobs. This idea sprang out of the Great Depression when Sidney Garfield, MD, had a small office near the Mojave Desert where there were many construction projects in operation. The lack of insurance companies meant fewer reimbursements, and when they were slow to pay, Dr. Garfield could not cover all of his expenses. One day Dr. Garfield's insurance agent recommended a pre-payment program. This program worked so well that it encouraged Dr. Garfield to create a larger health care program for his employees. He accepted a contract, with a workers' compensation program, for the Los Angeles aqueduct project in 1935. Then when he received a contract three years later to build the Grand Coulee Dam, he needed a way to handle the sicknesses and injuries of 6500 employees. During WWII he had government contracts to build ships in the San Francisco Bay Area community of Richmond. At the height of the war days he had over 90,000 employees. From these experiences, Dr. Garfield realized that the general public would be interested in this type of medical program, and so over the years he opened up his health care services, hospitals, and clinics, to several million people in various locations. In 1952 he changed the name of the medical program to Permanente Medical Group and established the Kaiser Foundation. Today they employ over 10,000 people and they have expansion plans. In addition, their Foundation focuses on meeting the needs of researchers with information relating to health care treatment, financing, administration, delivery, and the latest technologies, as well as social needs and interests. This vision covers prevention and self-help information, as well as research articles in support of social policies. Dr. Garfield was a strong leader who never asked what he could or could not do, thus he led by example, which is what the organizations he founded are practicing, and why they are held in high esteem by competitors, as well as public officials.

After WWII, companies began to pay employee benefits, such as health care and sick leave. Competition between companies focused on these benefits, as well as salary ranges, due to wage and price controls instituted during WWII. Physicians also had restraints on their prices, which were set by insurance companies as "usual, customary, and reasonable charges." By the 1950s most Americans came to expect health insurance coverage (Porter and Teisberg, 2006, p.73). As more and more people obtained health care insurance, some physicians raised their rates. Patients that did not like the higher rates would change to a different physician. Providers who want to raise their rates, cannot raise rates to those patients reimbursed by insurance; however, they can stop accepting certain insurance companies and instead accept cash, or they could even stop accepting all insurance and accept only cash. (This will be discussed further in Chapter Six). At this point, health care costs began to rise. Another factor in the rising costs included the availability of specialists, special equipment, testing, and specialized hospitals and health care services. Competition in health care has been increasing over the past fifty years and this is one of the major factors pushing reform.

Competition within the marketplace has traditionally been guarded and the company that sells the most gadgets will win awards and accolades within the industry journals. If you look at sports, in addition to players vs. management, and corporate management vs. industry leaders, there is fierce competition between players who may have some leverage over major league corporations, and sometimes competition between corporate management and local elected officials, who want the players of the teams to volunteer in local children's hospitals, advertise their car dealerships, or promote a major grocery store chain in the team's city. Without competition players seldom excel, team management pays the least amount they can, and then they lose players who refuse to take less.

As more dollars began flowing into the health care industry, outside forces jumped into health care to join the feeding frenzy. Corporations that traded on Wall Street found unlimited funding to build hospitals, both inpatient and outpatient, heliport pads on hospitals or clinics, and to buy more modern equipment. Thus, corner store convenience was not as important as making a profit; however, seldom do the big dollars reach the producers, or in other words, the providers. Insurance companies now tell the provider what they will have to accept or they will need to practice elsewhere. They can also tell the providers what forms to use and what equipment and procedures to bill for within that practice. To insure that their procedures are completed to their satisfaction, they can send auditors and/or case managers into a practice. This then takes up time and adds additional costs to the practice as provider and staff are forced to pull patient's charts from four or five years back, and then answer questions regarding those charts. These audits have increased significantly since 2011, when providers in private practice began to be targeted. Private practice providers are considered fee-for-service providers, which many states, such as Texas, are targeting. There is a push to force them out of private practice and into an Affordable Care Organization (ACO), that can be controlled easier by state governments.

In a manner of speaking, the health care industry became a teenager. We all know how turbulent and restless teenagers are, and the health care industry was no exception. The cottage industry of health care services was left behind in the 1950s and 1960s, which was when the golden age of building hospitals began and with it the beginning of the end for the typical private practice. Wall Street took note of the funding for mergers and the giant health care buildings and organizations that were spawning around the nation. Health maintenance organizations (HMOs) and managed care organizations (MCOs) followed Blue Cross and Blue Shield, have learned from them, and are now dominating the insurance industry.

> A health maintenance organization is an organization that provides or arranges managed care for health insurance, self-funded health care benefit plans, individuals, and other entities in the United States as a liaison with health care providers (hospitals, doctors, etc.) on a prepaid basis. The Health Maintenance Organization Act of 1973 required employers with 25 or more employees to offer federally certified HMO options if the employer offers traditional health care options. Unlike traditional indemnity insurance, an HMO covers care rendered by those doctors and other professionals who have agreed by contract to treat patients in accordance with the HMO's guidelines and restrictions in exchange for a steady stream of customers. HMOs cover emergency care regardless of the health care provider's contracted status (Dorsey, 1975, pp. 1-9).

This way of doing business in health care means that there will again be greater control on medical decision making and on what services will be accessible. For some who shy away from visiting a mental health provider, there is the lingering stigma of "I'm not crazy" (Corrigan, 2004, pp. 614-625). The "crazy" one is the person who suffers from anxiety and depression but refuses professional help. This fear and mistrust tends to interfere with the acceptance of anyone outside of the primary care physician. Teenagers and adults often note their apprehension with mental health diagnostic labels (Wright, 2011). The Institute of Medicine has estimated that over 18,000 Americans die prematurely each year, simply because they lack health insurance (Brownlee, 2007, p. 1).

An accessibility policy for over 40 million Americans is part of the Affordable Care Act of 2010. Anytime 40 million people enter the health care system, there will be chaos. There are several steps within this act that will culminate in 2014, when almost all Americans can be expected to have some health care coverage for the first time in America's history (See the next section – What This Means to Private Practice). One General Motors' executive told Senator Tom Daschle, "the high cost of health care is the single largest impediment to creating more jobs in the United States" (Daschle, 2008 p. 20). Part of the problem with getting consensus about what type of reform Americans want for health care is the multiphasic nature of change.

Congress, the President, and state governors are going to be facing more political pressure due to the shootings of five to seven year olds in a Newtown, Connecticut elementary school in December 2012. For weeks afterwards, twenty-four hours a day, seven days a week, we saw reports of the investigations, the burials, and how the tragedy affected people across the country; not just those living in Newtown. President Obama went to Newtown and spent time with the families and the first responders before addressing the nation in a news broadcast. From Roosevelt's fireside chats, to Nixon's "Checker" (his dog) chats, to Bill Clinton's town meetings, the way to communicate with America is to talk about what is on the minds of her people. One person claimed "the president's most powerful weapon...is a public aroused on a specific issue" (Miller, 1993, p. 314; Weissert and Weissert, 2002, p. 97). For providers to try to help fix many of the problems at the heart of their concern, they need to find, or create, a platform that will generate open discussions of how providers can become a united force and where their issues are once again addressed with them, instead of without them. This platform must also include building a political force such as a Super PAC (Chapter Two). The Super PAC is like a traditional PAC (Political Action Committee) without many of the restrictions. For instance, a Super PAC can raise and spend unlimited amounts of money for the sole purpose of supporting or opposing political candidates. Even so, after all the special interest groups have paraded in front of the camera, what are the chances that any meaningful event happens to reduce health care costs when hospitals are the centers of bulging costs, not private practices?

The health care industry is composed of a variety of components: providers, technology, pharmaceutical components, researchers, administrators, financiers, hospitals, insurance companies, specialties in legislative regulations, law enforcement agencies that include auditors, statisticians, and licensing boards. At the center of all these different components is the patient holding the gold, or silver, or paper insurance identification card.

During the 1970s there was an expansion of HMOs and MCOs. By the 1980s, insurance companies realized that their profits were shrinking and they did what any businessperson would do; they raised their premiums. When the corporations saw the dramatic rise in premiums they had to do what any businessperson would do; they passed it on to the consumer. When consumers complained with their feet, the big products stopped moving and car sales decreased. While the oil companies were increasing their premiums, other American companies did what every big corporation does and called their industry leaders, who called the American Chamber of Commerce, and everyone called their lobbyists, who then went to Congress and the state legislators. Congress approved a managed care system whose goal was to reduce premiums. Managed care was offered through managed care organizations (MCOs) and health maintenance organizations (HMOs). The HMOs fell out of favor with the general public, as well as with providers, because they were very aggressive in case management and utilization reviews. In other words, they denied services and coverage. People died and movies were made about HMOs and their practice of medicine.

WHAT DOES THIS MEAN TO PRIVATE PRACTICE?

Heath care is a business, something most providers have been putting aside for the last 25 years. Those who received degrees and licenses within the past twenty years have chosen the milieu by which to offer their services, i.e. within hospitals, outpatient services, non-profit organizations, military or government, industry, limited partnerships, and private practice. Since the introduction of the Affordable Care Act of 2010 the normal relationship of provider to insurer has begun to unwind, including the increased attention to law enforcement by insurers and Medicaid and Medicare administrators. At one time the private practitioner may have offered to see Medicaid patients at a flat rate above other rates, but these special arrangements have been left behind as providers are not seen as being in a position of strength to negotiate anything due to the ACT of 2010. The whole attitude has changed, and now insurers are the bullies on the block, "deal with it or get out," which has been witnessed in Texas. Whereas, in some states, such as Oregon, there have been efforts to work with providers in groups, and as a result hospitals and Affordable Care Organizations have received more power, money, and privileges that those in private practice lose.

Providers are the producers of health care services. In a normal marketplace producers are the ones who create the product or service that is sold to the public. There are many business-related steps that follow the creation process, such as doing a study on how a product or a service can be enhanced to make it more attractive to the public, as well as ways in which it can be more competitive against similar products and services. Defining that difference leads to a marketing scheme and has an effect on consumer choices. These features are the bells and whistles of a product or service. Also to consider when creating a product or service, is how to reduce the manufacturing cost in order to create a better profit margin. Features and profit margins go hand-in-hand. If the product or service is something that people need and want, but there are many competitors with similar products or services, then it has to be made more attractive to the customer. One way to do this is to keep the cost low. What makes it more attractive to the producer is the opportunity for profit. Not just any profit, but one that makes the provider a worthwhile return on their investment. In car sales, the owner of a franchise agrees to follow certain ethical standards of quality in service and sales that reflect favorably on the maker of the cars sold, as well as the entire automobile industry. The early providers of health care operated within the health care industry, which was in a cottage industry model at that time because no one knew how to harness the financial or the product/service side of the industry. As hospitals grew, demand grew for medical and allied services, such as physical therapy, occupational therapy, mental health services, chiropractic treatments, and nursing care.

For one group of providers operating during this time, their experience was similar to what is being experienced today. One former group member, a psychologist, reported:

> Over 25 years ago, I was a practicing psychotherapist as part of a team with psychiatry, psychology, and neurology at a very well respected private clinic. We had great freedom and we were empowered by our collaborative opportunity to support each other with the unique talents of our special training. Then the new concept of health maintenance organizations emerged and a growing presence of control over our practices came about, as you have outlined in your book. As a result, the clinic eventually disbanded as the professionals scattered becoming employees in the various HMO organizations, attempting to set up their own private practice or simply discontinuing their practice and retiring to something else. I attempted to create a counseling center offering a place for individual professional counselors to practice as independent contractors. That worked well for a short while but discontinued largely for economic reasons (Diehl, 2013).

Over the past dozen years MCOs dominated. Now, with the Affordable Care Act, HMOs are back. The combination of high costs, unsatisfactory quality, and limited access to health care has created anxiety and frustration for all participants. No one is happy with the current system – not patients, who worry about the cost of insurance and the quality of care; not employers, who face escalating premiums and unhappy employees; not physicians and other providers, whose incomes have been squeezed, professional judgments overridden, and workdays overwhelmed with bureaucracy and paperwork; not health plans, which are routinely vilified; not suppliers of drugs and medical devices, which have introduced many life-saving or life-enhancing therapies but get blamed for driving up costs; and not governments whose budgets are spinning out of control (Porter and Teisberg, 2006, p. 1).

This act was created because there was a change in policy in the White House. While policy makers do not live in the White House, they receive their directions from the President and his cabinet of advisors. They have chosen to make health care available to all American citizens, as well as those who have legal access to the American health care system. For a couple of years the policymakers, who came from a variety of disciplines and from all across the United States, held meetings. Other contributors to this policy development were from the academic arena, non-profit foundations, think tanks, such as Kaiser, Harvard, and Heritage Foundation, and a variety of corporate policy-making institutions. These are the organizations that publish books, journals, and articles that are read by decision makers. Being part of a policy-making organization or committee gives both the individual and the organization greater influence on the decision makers in the legislative branches of state and federal government similar to, but not in the same fashion as, lobbyists.

If a survey was taken of a representative of each component of the health care industry, one might not be surprised to learn that each component thinks they know what the patient wants, as well as what is best for the patient. For example, in the use of electronic hardware and software that is designed to share medical and mental health records between hospitals and medical and mental health care providers, there is a debate on the use of a universal ID number on all records called a universal patient identifier (UPI). Some doctors argue that this is the safest way to ensure that they have the right patient. Other doctors say that while this is a valid argument, it is also known that insurance companies have purchased lists of names in order to send out mailers to solicit business for health care, mortgage, credit card, and car insurance. Therefore, discussing only these two concerns demonstrates how two rational people can have different interpretations of the value of a product or service, and instead of increasing confidentiality, there is less today than before the Health Insurance Portability and Accountability Act (HIPAA) went into effect (Collins and Peel, 2012).

In discussing the effects of health care reform over the past 25 years, including issues of privacy and confidentiality, providers, as well as the general public, cannot ignore seven problems that continue to linger. In the rush to form HMOs to compete for the states' Medicaid populations, there has been a variety of interference between the components of the health care industry. The HMOs are public, for-profit corporations with stocks traded on Wall Street. Texas was one state that sent bids to several HMOs for a number of regions that were carved out of the Texas Medicaid population. This devolution of responsibility for social programs from the federal government to the states has its roots within the past three decades. This process focuses primarily on health care, income security, job training, and social services (Hurley and Wallin, 1998). More recently the federal government, through the Centers of Medicare and Medicaid Services (CMS), has established a State Resource Center (SRC) to centralize information about CMS state relations in an easily accessible format. In addition, this section of their website will house Medicaid data and systems information to assist state Medicaid agencies and researchers with their work relating to the Medicaid and CHIP programs (State Resource Center, 2012).

> Federal law also requires states to cover certain mandatory eligibility groups, which includes qualified parents, children, pregnant women, older adults, and those with disabilities with low incomes. States have the flexibility to cover

other optional eligibility groups and to set eligibility criteria within the federal standards. The Affordable Care Act of 2010 creates a new national Medicaid minimum eligibility level that covers most Americans with household income up to 133 percent of the federal poverty level. This new eligibility requirement is effective January 1, 2014, but states may choose to expand coverage before this date (State Resource Center, 2012).

According to this website, Medicaid's goals for 2013 are to:

- Increase access to affordable care; improving care and lowering costs; improve access to preventive services in Medicaid (effective January 1, 2013)
- Increase access to affordable care; increase Medicaid payments for primary care physicians (effective January 1, 2013 increments over time until December 31, 2014)

According to this website Medicaid's goals for 2014 are to:

- Increase access to affordable health care: create a system of affordable health care coverage (effective January 1, 2014)
- Improve access to affordable care; permit hospitals to make presumptive eligibility determinations (Effective January 1, 2014)

According to this website Medicaid's goals for 2015 are to:

- Improve access to affordable care; increase the federal matching rate for the Children's Health Insurance Program (effective October 1, 2015)

While the early signs of change in health care began with the introduction of Medicare and Medicaid during President Johnson's term in the 1960s, a decade later there were changes instituted in how hospitals were built, and in the 1980s, psychiatric hospitals began expanding. In order to regulate newly graduated personnel in mental health, licensing boards were also expanding. With licensing came recognition of professional degrees and of the ability to receive insurance reimbursement. State licensing boards focus on public accountability as well as policies, guidelines, and practices of medical, mental health, social work, and other professional boards deemed appropriate per each state. "In doing so, the book underscores the role of the Federation of State Medical Boards in facilitating state-based licensure and discipline and the promotion of quality health care" (Johnson and Chaudhry, 2012). During the 1980s when psychiatric hospitals began expanding, a 30-day inpatient treatment program for substance abuse was created, and then other inpatient treatments were created as co-dependency groups and depression groups. As physicians and allied providers learned about the new programs, hospitals received referrals from the allied providers, not just physicians. When transportation became a problem for some patients, outside sources contracted with hospitals to transport them. This escalated to the point that these hospitals were packed with patients, and when too much began to get too expensive and money began to fly off the charts, events occurred that brought the program to a screeching halt. This occurred in San Antonio, Texas when a 14-year old boy, who was living with his grandparents, was taken from his home and placed in Colonial Hills Psychiatric Hospital where he stayed for several days without seeing his physician. When his grandparents tried to sign him out, they were rebuffed, so they called their state representative, who was also an attorney (Stevens, 2009, p. 3; Willet, 2009). He got a habeas corpus form, law enforcement officials served the paper on the hospital, and as a result, the grandparents took him home. Not long after the court papers were served, a lengthy lawsuit began against the hospital, the psychiatrist (who did not have a valid Texas medical license), and the corporation that owned the hospital. From that point on, insurance organizations refused payments to all psychiatric hospitals, and the doors began to close. Problem One: greedy physicians and psychiatric hospitals; Problem Two: insurance companies becoming gatekeepers; Problem Three: many providers see the uneven playing field, as well as other problems within their profession, but act as if they are powerless to change it; Problem Four: therapists are not trained in the business side of therapy.

Doctors, as well as other health care providers, are notoriously poor business managers. Perhaps this began when providers focused on comforting, listening, and providing quality care for their patients. Today very few graduate schools offer any type of business courses for health care providers. Medical schools have taken the lead, nursing schools have followed, but mental health graduate programs have not, simply because there are very few psychologists who have experience in the business side of therapy and who are also professors in a graduate program. Therefore, those graduating with a degree in the mental health field do not understand the major or minor issues of the business side of providing care. In addition, providers of all health care disciplines have traditionally been like sheep, following a leader or a theorist, and not willing to take preventive measures to address the health care reform's repercussions on their practices. Very few have run for political office. Blame for an apathetic attitude toward the health care reform movement lies with many people, including psychiatrists and psychologists, who see each other as competitors rather than partners, choosing to chase each other around "issues" through letters to an editor or through articles in professional associations (Hixson, 2011, pp. 119-127). Signs of apathy include fatigue, answering in a curt fashion, anger, depression, and withdrawal from normal social activities. Psychiatrists are apprehensive of psychologists who have prescription pads and prescription rights for certain medications. Psychologists are separating themselves from non-doctorate level therapists by calling them "non-something,"; licensed therapists are discovering that the state is funding projects that create unfair competition for their private practices. For example, non-profit organizations form community mental health agencies or rural health care agencies and then receive grant funding from state and federal programs. Non-profit agencies have taken advantage of these grants to provide the 3,000 hours needed in licensing. In the case of mental health and mental retardation (MHMR) organizations, they have developed their own qualified mental health profession (QMHP) title (Friendship Development Services, 2008). Those who earn this certification, or designation, earn it with on-the-job training but in most cases they must have a bachelor's degree before the application is accepted. The grant-funded agencies obtain funding from Medicaid, as well as grants from charitable foundations and from the Department of Health and Human Services (DHHS). This allows them to train those who do not have a graduate degree or other health care license to consult with patients and to offer treatment at a lower cost. State insurance commissions have allowed non-profits to charge a flat fee for each individual they see per day. Others may use a fee schedule that is approved by an oversight commission.

Apathy is a lack of awareness in regards to common business terms and how they can be applied to a practice; it also describes the attitude of providers of various disciplines in health care services when it comes to business and politics.

Overhead expenses include the entire expense of running an office, such as office rent or mortgage, utilities, phone, computers, software, fax machine, shredder, copy paper, answering service, income taxes, property taxes, federal taxes, accounting fees, legal fees, professional association and licensing renewal fees, payroll, insurance, postage, forms, surveys or educational tools, advertising, bank fees, loan fees, marketing, recoupment, audit costs, storage costs, professional liability insurance, and professional convention(s) with travel costs. In order to determine how much money is needed to meet the monthly budget, monthly expenses should be added up and divided by 160 hours. This is the amount each hour should be billed. If the monthly budget is $16,000 then the hourly billing rate must be $100 per hour x 8 hours x 20 days. Most therapists have difficulty in reaching that rate, so as a result, they take a lower salary.

"No shows" cost practices lots of money each year, as do slow paying MCOs and HMOs (Chapter Four). If the billing rate is $50 per hour and only five patients are seen on an average day, then the budget is $5000, minus the slow payers who will drag out a reimbursement for two to four months, even though the practice must continue to keep the business running.

Sharing an office can help lower monthly budgets, but this could lower a physician's salary after making payments for education, certification, and licensing requirements for the new position. Welcome to the harsh reality of business! We are not missionaries, unless a church is supporting our practice. Too often we get into this profession because we want to help others; not because of the money. Taking an oath of poverty hurts your family and leads to a drop in energy, increasing frustration, and self-inflicted pity (Cummings and O'Donohue, 2008, pp. 139-163; Hixson, 2011, pp. 17-33). The apathy boils into hostility and defensiveness.

Private practitioners are having their reimbursement rates reduced to less than the amount needed for overhead expenses, while non-profits receive twice as much per hour than most mental health providers. For example, in border communities the rates are below costs of operation. Psychologists have taken a 30% hit over the past two years and are now being asked to take further cuts in addition to providing HMOs with more documentation. Master therapists are in the same boat; however, the rate of reimbursement is 30% BELOW psychologists. Their private practices are not 30% lower than psychologists. As a result, rural communities are losing treatment for mental health as these mental health providers close their offices and either turn to other careers, take an early retirement, or attempt to find work in another state. Texas is the lowest and Texas leads the nation in uninsured citizens with one in four residents not having insurance. In addition, Texas pays one of the lowest rates per child for education. In the author's community LPCs have been receiving calls to join an HMO or traditional Medicaid as providers. The LPCs in this border community all work for an education institution and have heard the horrendous stories happening to those who have had practices in this community for years. Now, if people need a psychologist or therapist they must travel over 150 miles to San Antonio. Since Medicaid and Medicare patients normally have fewer dollars to spend, transportation becomes problematic. Even if Medicaid authorizes it, there is a waiting list for transportation and another waiting list, of several months, to receive an appointment in San Antonio.

Primary care physicians (PCPs) are finding that Medicaid is refusing to pay for co-payments to Medicare policies, and Medicare is having doctors charge-off the first $500 dollars a year for each Medicare patient before they start paying the physician. These examples of inequities in reimbursement and practice creates its own storm of turmoil. Given the enormous pressure put on legislators in Congress by the American Medical Association (AMA), there was a statement issued through Kaiser Family Foundation:

> Medicaid fees for primary care services in 2013 will increase by 73%, on average, and will more than double in New York, California, Florida, and three other states under an endangered provision of the Affordable Care Act (ACA), according to a new study issued December 17 by the Kaiser Family Foundation.

The ACA boosts notoriously low Medicaid rates to Medicare levels in 2013 and 2014 for evaluation and management (E/M) services and vaccine administration for family physicians, general internists, pediatricians, and subspecialists related to these fields, such as pediatric cardiologists. Lawmakers included the pay hike to encourage physicians to accept more Medicaid patients in 2014, when states are scheduled to broaden eligibility requirements. Many states are choosing not to do so in the wake of this year's Supreme Court decision on the ACA that essentially made participation in Medicaid expansion voluntary (Lowes, 2012).

The Texas Medical Association's 47,000 physicians took a day off in early 2013 to protest what they described as "a harm to access to care for thousands of dual-eligible patients who qualify for Medicare and Medicaid" (Health, 2013, p. 4A). According to the article, doctors were refusing to see new dual-eligible patients while others have stopped accepting Medicare and Medicaid patients. Victor Gonzalez, MD was quoted as saying that "he exhausted his personal savings of $50,000 and took out bank loans so he could keep his doors open to continue to care for the people of his community (South Texas border) (p.4a). It is estimated that this would affect over 320,000 people in Texas.

Some physicians argue that the "good old days" are gone within private practice. Providers of all disciplines are losing patients after a new HMO or MCO takes over the management of patient care in a region. Dentists have reported that they have lost up to half of their practices because their practice was not approved for a position on their list of practice panels. Chiropractors have complained that they have a hard time gaining HMOs and MCOs panel access. A panel is a position on their list of qualified providers. To be on the panel, they must have completed their paperwork and have been accepted as a provider for the company. Physical therapists need a referral from the PCP. Podiatrists and occupational therapists have also seen a significant drop in case loads since the HMOs capture of Medicaid contracts. Many mental health providers are closing their private practices, while others are going into case management (a gatekeeper position with HMOs), or sharing office space with another provider, some are returning to school for another degree, or accepting positions within non-profit organizations, a governmental position, or a job with the Veterans Administration.

PCPs are pulling out of Medicaid and/or Medicare programs because their reimbursement rates are below costs. Some PCPs are refusing any new Medicaid or Medicare patients, others are retiring early, and some are accepting teaching positions. The shortage of physicians and mental health care providers continues to grow unabated. While providers may see more patients after 2014, the treatment plan or their approach to helping families was the primary reason for patients to return as needed. With the influx of new eligible patients in 2014, their HMO will refer them and it will not be by the provider's reputation. This is an important issue with providers who have practiced for many years. Personal and professional identity as well as pride in their skills is being challenged, and they, as others before them, are sensing that it is time to reconsider their professional goals. An example of this are the doctors who have basically turned their practices over to physician assistants (PAs) and have gone fishing because they have been working long days for so long that they didn't always feel human, unless it was to feel a patient's pain. Other providers reflect on their experiences over the past several years and reveal how the "fun" has gone of their practices.

Another group that is having problems with Medicaid and the Attorney General's office is the Physician Assistants who have opportunities to purchase a practice from a retiring physician. Here is one story from Texas:

In June of 2011, the Physician Assistant Political Alliance (PAPA) was created by a coalition of physician assistant leaders in response to the passage of House Bill 2098. It now exists as a sovereign organization with its sole interest to protect and improve the practice environment of Texas' physician assistants and also to represent our profession to health policy leaders.

House Bill 2098, which passed in the last legislative session, was worded in such a fashion that it made it unlawful for physician assistants to own more than 49% of a practice or to have any official capacity or control of a practice they jointly own with a physician. Specifically, a physician assistant could not be an officer or a board member of the business entity even if they were the driving force in developing it. The bill was not retroactive and existing clinics were, therefore, grandfathered. PAPA was created to work to undo the adverse effects the bill created. In the spring of 2012 the Texas Medical Board (TMB) adopted the language of HB 2098 into its rules and added additional language that should the ownership interest in these grandfathered clinic businesses ever change, then that business entity would become subject to the new board rules. Further, the board asked all physician assistants with business interests in their practices to file with the board and to sign a legal agreement that they agreed to this new rule imposing restraints on physician assistant businesses.

The Physician Assistant Business Alliance of Texas (PABAT) was subsequently formed as an inclusive entity for physician assistants, not wishing to be named litigants, to file suit against the Texas Medical Board after the TMB rule was adopted. Their position was to argue that the board acted outside its rule-making authority. There was no fundamental agreement that the board had any jurisdiction over the business practices of physician assistants. The board is tasked with licensing and disciplining medical providers, thereby protecting the public, and is not tasked as a business bureau subrogating the office of the Texas Secretary of State.

On September 11th, 2012, a district court ruling agreed with PAPAT and PAPA. The Attorney General's office and the Texas Medical Board had thirty days to appeal the ruling. On the last day for an appeal, Friday, October 19th, 2012, the TMB filed an appeal challenging the judicial outcome.

To summarize, the Court's findings that were favorable to physician assistants are as follows:

- HB 2098 is meant to apply only to entities jointly owned by a physician assistant and a physician. It does not apply to business entities solely owned by physician assistants.
- For jointly owned entities, HB 2098's restrictions are not triggered when a physician assistant contracts with a new supervising physician. (Importantly, this ruling provides case law that supports the ability of physician assistants to contract physicians as medical directors.)
- HB 2098's grandfather clause continues to apply to all co-owned entities that existed prior to June 17, 2011, as long as there is no change in any ownership interest in the entity.
- The law actively discourages physician assistants from partnering with physicians.
- A physician assistant—even one who was not a part of the suit— can hire a supervising physician so long as they are not in a non-grandfathered, jointly owned entity.

HB 2098 is completely inapplicable to a physician assistant solely owned entity.

Another group that has been hit hard is the family pharmacies. One pharmacist offered the following as an example of how small pharmacies are hurt by the current health care reform.

> This is one story about the death of the independent pharmacies. When I graduated in 1993 from the University of Texas at Austin, School of Pharmacy, I was told that the future of independent pharmacies was soon coming to an end. I believed this for the first six years of my career, while working for Wal-mart. A seasoned pharmacist of over 50 years tried yearly to get me to purchase his independent pharmacy. One day I took him up on his offer, since I wanted something more out of my awesome profession. I soon learned that not only were independent pharmacies not dead, they offered opportunities to make my profession into a great career. Mixing medicine and business was exciting to me. I would soon learn that an independent pharmacist could have more freedom to interact with their customers and patients could be more accessible to them, and more importantly, cater to their individual needs. I soon learned that big chain pharmacies actually made independent pharmacies shine, due to the poor service they gave to these same customers. I could now focus on the patient and their medical needs. Whatever they needed; medicine,

help with insurance, special needs or anything that would help them obtain better health, I could do it because I wanted to help by providing this service.

The seasoned pharmacist would come and check on me from time to time and would ask me how I was able to take the payments from the large company insurances, especially since what they paid the pharmacist was below what it actually cost to provide the medicine or service. I told him that it was all a numbers game, large volume mixed with the right population of customers, such as those with Medicaid, which meant most of our elderly and children, are being insured by the government. These were the people that needed the services of the independent pharmacist the most, and we were being somewhat compensated for assisting this population of customers. The numbers added up and I felt I could make a living doing what I loved doing best while also investing my profits into opening two other strategically placed pharmacies. I was excited to recruit younger pharmacists, hometown kids and graduates to come back home and help their community. Not only did I have to convince them that it was the best move for them, but I also had to back it up by paying them what a big chain pharmacy would pay them.

Within four years of opening my first store, I would have three strong pharmacies with 30 full time and part time employees. I was able to give back to the community, not only with great pharmacy service, but I was also able to contribute to charitable organizations and school scholarships, as the major pharmacies do, without thinking twice. The times were good for a while, as I thanked my lucky stars that I made such a move early in my profession. Things would soon change as Medicare part D would come into play. A plan by the government was created to allow senior citizens to participate in a drug medication play. Unfortunately for independent pharmacies, this was a government plan that would be run by HMO's and large private insurances. Not only did this plan allow for senior citizens to have access to such drug plans, which I felt was a great idea in theory, but it allowed for senior citizens that were on a state run program, like Medicaid, to also be placed on this plan. Now what seemed so simple and perfect was the beginning of the end for independent pharmacies. We were now forced to take on new contracts in order to provide service for our customers. The transition from state Medicaid to Medicare part D was a nightmare in itself. The confusion and the unorganization would test the limits of all pharmacies, whether big or small. It caused a panic among the elderly who could not access their refills or medications at the pharmacy of their choice, and in some cases Medicaid patients were forced to take plans that were not taken by their own pharmacy. Pharmacists were forced to choose between trying to help the patient by giving them their medication or waiting for clarification as to what plan would pay for their medication.

I cannot speak for all independent pharmacists, but I can speak for most pharmacists and myself in my underserved area, that we gave them the medications without payment. We lost thousands during that time. We all knew that we had no choice; we couldn't leave our customers, friends, neighbors, and relatives in the cold. We did what was right and what was necessary. We would end up losing a lot of customers that year, mainly because we didn't participate in some of the larger chains preferred insurances. There was a reason we didn't accept those insurances in the first place; not only were they paying low reimbursements, but these third parties also encouraged our customers to use their mail order service. Not to mention not paying for all the services those independent pharmacies provided, like delivery or on call services. Eventually I was forced to choose between taking a horrible insurance in order to keep the customer or to let them go. As a businessman, I knew that you couldn't give more out than you take in. It would just be a matter of time before something would give. That something would be the privatization of the Texas run Medicaid drug program. It was not a great idea to give this program to the big insurance companies, but it would also affect the people that needed it the most: those in the most underserved areas of this great state of Texas. Because of a budget shortfall, where everything was being cut, pharmacies seemed to get the brunt of the cut. I would personally take the time out of my workday and money out of my pocket to attend and to even speak to different congressional panels, about the importance of what independent pharmacies do. It must have fallen on deaf ears, because the Medicaid program was privatized and like déjà vu, the hardest hit was our poor, disabled, elderly and children that all needed the services of the independent pharmacy. Like in Medicare part D, pharmacies were forced to either take an insurance plan in order to serve their already existing customers or lose their customers. Like history repeating itself, independent pharmacies were forced to take on the challenge of giving medication and services without reimbursements, while insurance companies were adjusting to these new customers. Thousands of dollars were lost again, but this time the wounds weren't healing. What used to sustain a modest independent pharmacy was no longer enough to allow the pharmacy to stay in business. Each pharmacy made adjustments to try to survive, such as cuts in staff, donations, inventory, expenses, hours, and service. The end was near, as independent pharmacy after independent pharmacy was closing. No waving white flag, no letter of surrender; just a quick painful deathblow to the heart of independent pharmacies all across the state, mine included. Like the captain of a sinking ship, who is either the last to get off or he goes down with his ship, I slowly let people go, after their years of service and loyalty. The pain was in everyone's eyes, customers, patients, staff, and family, the end had arrived.

Larger pharmacies, such as Wal-Mart, Walgreens, CVS, Rite Aid, Kroger, Target, and Kaiser Permanente, have the economy of scale and can provide margins of profit, which independent pharmacies cannot due to the difference in volume of customers. Home health agencies are on the cutting block, too. Here is a comment from one independent owner.

My family opened our company in January 2008 and we received our provider number in November 2010 due to their waiting period. All services provided during that period were not reimbursable. It was a long struggle and we are proud of what we have accomplished. My company is small with 12 employees and we cover four rural border counties at the present time. Now we are threatened with the reform, which promises drastic cuts in reimbursable services and reimbursements for all home health agencies. Reimbursements will be lower and more difficult to collect. Visits will be minimized and some supplies will not be covered. The company will still be responsible for providing the highest level of care with minimal financial assistance from the private insurance/government. Since every insurance company has their own rates, there is no set fee; therefore, your company may receive an overpayment invoice, or recoupment, and the insurer demands their money back within 15 days. How is it possible to know if it's overpaid, if there are no published rates? How can your business grow if you're struggling, with no way to communicate with someone who can help you improve, or at least understand the system better? Home health agencies have a lot of expenses that are required in order to receive full payment such as, yearly cost reports, billing, monthly surveys with the IRS and Texas Workforce Commission. Then we are responsible to our employees and we have the costs of overhead expenses of our office space. With the promised cuts, I don't see how I can survive. Then what happens to the patients?

Therapy and physician groups in Texas have been alarmed for two years since they first learned about the cuts and other changes in the delivery of health care services. According to a Ft. Worth newspaper dated November 20, 2011, the state had already earmarked over $150 million dollars to be cut from therapists who treat patients in Texas per year. For those therapists in speech, occupational, physical, and mental health, this led to reimbursement rates anywhere from 30% to 71% for each procedure. Patients ask what happened to their old plan; their provider? Why were they switched to another primary care physician or why did they lose their psychiatrist? Some patients, who have relied on Medicaid transportation or funding to travel an hour or more to a provider, have now lost those benefits. Psychologists now have waiting periods from eight to ten months and some psychiatrists have waiting periods for more than 12 months. These changes translate into: a loss of accessibility to timely health care services; time can be important in the delivery of quality health care; and psychological evaluations are common in the diagnostic process of a mental health evaluation. It can ferret out critical pieces of information that can change a treatment plan and/or educational goals and plans. The consequences include depriving students of a special education program for lack of adequate documentation. Even speech therapists have stopped treating some children because of a change in coverage by the new insurance provider. These changes invite the question: what is pushing health care practice in this new reformation—costs or medical and/or mental health needs? MCOs and HMOs are taking control of who can bill for their covered population and they are dictating more procedures and limitations to the providers and the patients as we get closer to January 1, 2014.

Rural communities are normally the last area in any state to gain adequate health care. For example, border communities along the Mexican border have problems not faced by border communities with Canada. A rural community between El Paso, Texas and Laredo, Texas covers about 2000 miles. In this area there are three psychologists, no psychiatrists, 29 licensed professional counselors and one social worker. In this area, according to Border Statistics, there are 30% more seniors than the average county in Texas, twice the number of Hispanics of origin, twice the number of Spanish speaking people, and 70% more that fall below the poverty level. Compare these figures to the number of therapists in Travis County, which includes the city of Austin; there are 990 square miles and in this area there are 139 psychologists, 150 psychiatrists, 244 licensed professional counselors, and 144 social workers. One psychologist, who has worked in a border community for over 20 years, has been watching as both Medicaid and Medicare reimbursement rates have tumbled over the past five years. From the wife of a psychologist came this note:

> Reviewing our past five years of actual financial data makes an irrefutable argument to close our outpatient practice. We have been discussing creating an exit strategy for termination thereof; however, we are in a quandary because for years my husband has been the only doctoral level mental health practitioner who is a Medicaid/Medicare provider in our region, which is quite large. In fact, if he is unable to go to work on any given day, he has no backup coverage. The overheads are killing us along with the no show rate. We cannot bill Medicaid patients for their failure to show for a scheduled appointment, so that becomes our "opportunity cost" foregone. And of course, the reimbursement cutbacks from Medicare/Medicaid and others have taken a bite. Our overheads continue to rise and employees expect annual raises, bonuses, and other perks, which means the only one who absorbs the reduced cash flow is the doctor. Over the past five years, I have averaged $8k per annum via W2 compensation for myself. Meanwhile, as a MBA graduate, I could be holding down a regular, well-paying job that would probably have medical benefits. We are unable to obtain any type of company health coverage because we are so small. Keeping up with the demands created by the outpatient practice consume a tremendous amount of my time: proofing intakes, reviewing billing reports (aged receivables, etc.), denials on claims, all the contracting paperwork for the MCOs, EFT setup, running payroll, taking care of invoices, keeping the books (Quick-Books), and ordering supplies. There is not a day goes by where we do not have to write a letter to a PCP or to a school; we are always getting SSI paperwork for folks looking to get the disability cash flow. Parents of a high percentage of children that are new patients end up submitting for SSI Disability (about 90%). When my husband gets home at night, he is drained.

> Our commercial revenues have been running less than 5% of our total. Unlike metropolitan areas, there is no way to compensate for sub-par reimbursement rates with a solid commercial mix. Further, there is no governmental compensation for the extensive travel, which is part of living and working in a medically underserved area (MUA) to get to the nursing homes that so badly need

these services. Worse, ironically Medicare reimbursement rates are lower for rural areas in Texas. The cost of living may be lower in the rural areas, but the cost of doing business is higher. The last two years (2011 and 2012) were both "in the red" for the outpatient business (OP). Even in his highest OP revenue year, he could have earned over $63 per hour more had he worked at the NH, since he would not have been burdened with high overheads and additional staff. I hope that we close the OP practice, but if and when is up to my husband. The financial decision is easy, but the personal one is not. Herb feels obligated both to doctors and to patients, and he hates to lay people off, so this is a very difficult decision for him to make. He knows that many of the patients, who really need mental health services, will "go without" because they do not have the means to travel to San Antonio, Laredo, San Angelo, etc. to get like-kind services. Local mental health and mental retardation is a joke. I hear they only use a psychiatrist via TeleMed.

From a psychologist who works in a community where the hospital is purchasing physician practices in order to build a medical home with the ACO model comes an observation:

I've been working for a year trying to coordinate with the hospital and the group of psychologists and licensed professional counselors (LPCs) and social workers in this county, but the hospital wants to pay the LPCs and social workers $25 an hour and psychologists $35 an hour. There is no good alternative for mental health providers. I've spent over $100,000 on my education, then another $80,000 over the past 15 years building up my practice. I cannot sell it and I'm going to lose it because the patients will go to the hospital's program.

The shortages of providers have led to access problems within health care services, which is incongruent with the stated goals of the Affordable Care Act (Act) of 2010. By 2014 millions of new eligible patients, who presently have no health care policy or coverage, will be eligible for Medicaid coverage. States that have recruited insurance companies to bid on the Medicaid population are preparing for an inflated budget in 2014 and 2015 that will have to be addressed. It would seem like the states, who are struggling to balance state budgets, see an opportunity to go through a loophole in the Act in order to control their costs of the millions of new providers. Without access, there are fewer bills against Medicaid. Blue Cross Blue Shield of Oregon, through their Regency Policy, is able to deny mental health services to patients if they belong to a group policy that has less than 50 enrollees, which would also include those that purchase policies independent of a group.

Problem Six: providers are dropping out of the field or leaving private practice to work for non-profit organizations, government or educational institutions, or joining an ACO, or some are even changing careers (Hogg

Foundation, 2012; Human Resources Services Administration, 2012; George, 2011).

Physician shortages have been with us for decades, especially in the mental health field. Now we see shortages in physicians, especially primary care physicians (Elliott, 2012). "Only 36% of practicing physicians will hold a practice ownership stake by the end of the 2013, down from 57% in 2000, according to Accenture's analysis of data from the American Medical Association and MGMA-ACMPE". Nurses are overcoming shortages, but more nurses are required to be given additional responsibilities in the mental health field, HMO and MCO case management, audits, or utilization reviews. Going back a decade:

> About two-thirds of primary care physicians (PCPs) reported in 2004–05 that they could not get outpatient mental health services for patients—a rate that was at least twice as high as that for other services. Shortages of mental health care providers, health plan barriers, and lack of coverage or inadequate coverage were all cited by PCPs as important barriers to mental health care access. The probability of having mental health access problems for patients varied by physician practice, health system, and policy factors. The results suggest that implementing mental health parity nationally will reduce some, but not all, of the barriers to mental health care (Cunningham, 2009).

The parity movement was championed in Congress by Paul Wellstone, Pete Domenici, Senator Ted Kennedy, and Presidents Carter and Clinton, and this effort and support led to the Mental Health Parity and Addiction Equity (MHPAE) Act of 2008. This Act was to eliminate differences in insurance coverage for behavioral health. Mental health and addiction treatment advocates have long viewed parity as a means of increasing fairness in the insurance market, and also for opening greater access to mental health care treatment. Corporate employers, HMOs, and MCOs have opposed it because of concerns about costs. The costs they are often talking about are earmarked for their pockets, including bonuses. They have a vested interest in cutting accessibility and benefits.

> The system giveth and the system taketh away. It takes your money, time, health, and it gives generously to Wall Street and fat-cat businesspeople and hospital executives who earn millions of dollars. Dr. William W. McGuire, the former CEO of United Health Care, one of the country's largest health consumers, not only received $1.7 billion worth of stock options during his tenure, but also had a jet at his disposal and a red carpet reportedly rolled out to meet his limo so his tootsies did not have to meet the same ground on which we ordinary mortals step. This money, or at least some of it, could have provided better health care or lower costs for United Health Care's enrollees, but instead it wound up in Dr. McGuire's very large bank account and literally fell under his feet (Herzlinger, 2007, pp. 15-16).

The conclusion of most MCOs and HMOs is that the value of health care services is not the ability to understand the symptomology of an illness or disorder, or to treat the pain, disease, or disorder effectively, but to treat it more efficiently; in other words, by reducing access and treatment, they lower the costs of health care. Taking reimbursement dollars from the providers, who are the creators of health and wellbeing in most cases, and giving it to MCOs or HMOs in order to manage providers and cases, creates a trade from Peter to Paul. State legislators and state health and insurance commissions are now taking the initiative to change health care practices by changing the administrative system of reimbursement and case management. They are doing this primarily to control state health care expenditures and to balance state budgets. Therefore, the administrators of the health care plans are more important to the budget because they have the authority to say how much is paid for services, what services can be reimbursed, and how often or how much will be allotted for specialty care including long term care. Now when MCOs or HMOs deny claims, or interfere with access, they are saving the state money and this results in a bonus for their own corporation. While at one time the providers had these roles and responsibilities, now people without a health care license or educational degree in a health care discipline are calling the shots, and they have the influence from the governor and the attorney general to perform such roles. This is called "corporate practice of medicine."

> The traditional health care system, dominated by the professional guild and financed by indemnity insurance, has been shattered beyond any possibility of repair. Once complacent taxpayers and formerly paternalistic employers have fought back against inflating costs and escalating premiums, choking back the once massive flow of subsidies for inefficient small practices, fragmented delivery systems, and cost-unconscious consumer demand. We observe turbulent cycles of expansion and contraction, diversification and refocusing, mergers and divestitures; however, the system never returns to the status quo ante. The emerging organization of medicine will resemble neither the cottage industry of professional dominance nor the vertically integrated system of managed competition (Robinson, 1999, pp.211-212).

One physician who had a private practice, then became the medical director of a clinic, and then the medical director of an HMO, saw firsthand how managed care chases the dollar, not in order to balance budgets, but to make a profit, something they blame fee-for-service providers for doing.

> Until we remove the motive of profit from financing of health care, we will not solve the health care crisis. Any group that proposes reform policy that maintains the use of for-profit insurance companies in a so-called free market is being driven by a single motive – to protect the golden coffers of their share of the $2 trillion cash cow! (LeBow, 2007, p. xvii).

Profits and greed have been yanked away from providers and turned over to the HMOs and MCOs. By using the argument that health care costs are too high, government officials have distracted the public from the issues of corporate greed in HMOs and MCOs. They have an incentive to slow down reimbursements, to charge providers with over payments, and to deny benefits.

Problem Seven: greedy HMOs and MCOs. There is at least one person who thinks that this is a good time for physicians to open up a private practice. That person is not a physician, but she has a lot of experience in health care, particularly working with coding, billing, and administration. She writes that she is a:

> Certified Professional Coder and is Board Certified in Medical Practice Management and a Fellow in the American College of Medical Practice Executives. My partner, Abraham Whaley, has 15+ years of experience in patient access, registration, patient/family customer service, quality assurance, and information technology in private physician groups and emergency medicine/hospital settings (Whaley, 2012).

According to Pat Whaley here are five good reasons to start a PCP in 2013:

- The demand overshadows the supply now and in 2014 it is expected to be at least 15% + greater depending on where the office is opened.
- Fractional practice administrators (FPA) are available to assist new practices getting started and to stay on the right track. Once started, an FPA may only be needed one hour a week.
- The cost of an EMR/EHR is no longer a barrier to the private physician.
- Attaining a retiring physician's practice does not need to be the costly proposition as in the past.

Someone else suggests that the trend with PCPs, at least in Wyoming, is leaving private practice and working in a hospital with a group of physicians. Some hospitals have purchased practices, but the reader may need to address this issue directly with the hospital administrator.

> The trend is happening in Cheyenne too, as more doctors are joining the staff of Cheyenne Regional Medical Center through its Cheyenne Regional Physicians Group. Doctors say joining a hospital's staff enables them to focus on medicine without worrying about the business headaches. The trend shows 50% of physicians in many communities work for the hospital. In just two years it is predicted that hospitals will account for more than 75% of all new doctor hires in America, Merritt Hawkins reports. Five years ago, about 25% of the country's doctors were employed by hospitals or large physician businesses, said Dr. John Lucas, chief executive officer at Cheyenne Regional Medical Center (Orr, 2012).

In summary, one man's junk is another's gold mine. Timing, location, having a good business plan, having some money to put into the project, or having a co-signer or investor, preferably someone with experience in starting up a practice or business, are all necessary ingredients of a business proposal. Physicians, generally speaking, are just as naive as psychologists, psychotherapists, physical therapists, and chiropractors when it comes to preparing a business plan or a proposal for financing. Thirty years ago these skills were never considered necessary to the education process for health care providers. Today it is.

History teaches us that when we fail to remember the lessons of the past, we are committing ourselves to repeating our mistakes. History matters because it can teach us of the future. As discussed earlier, the issues of change are not just with a system of administration or financing, but it is a system of accessibility and delivery. Up to this point government has chosen to use surrogates to do their dirty work. Over the past 30 years, Wall Street corporations have learned from this experience and are using their unique position to control the bottom line. They are using state regulations, state law enforcement, and federal contacts and support agreements to perform in ways that would appear, in the global marketplace, as illegal. The basic concept states that patients may have the right to choose their PCP, but the PCP can thwart them by a law of competition in the region, or by a lack of cooperation, or other regulations built in to allow the HMO to change their provider accidentally or for administrative purposes. Legislatures pass laws that legislators seldom read or fully understand, which explains why some legislators say they are supportive of quality health care, but then vote for legislation that hampers quality in health care delivery.

Practitioners are feeling left out of the equation due to the fact that decisions are being made that affect their practices both directly and indirectly and leaves them without any control over their practice. Therefore, they are voting with their feet and leaving the state or even leaving the field by taking an early retirement. When all the new eligible patients come to a state like Texas, they will find long lines and overworked providers. Rick Perry said it best in a February 2013 interview: "Why should I extend Medicaid? I don't have enough providers." Well said, Mr. Governor. Now who is responsible for that?

In the next chapter we will discover what the fight is over. The rabbit is chasing its carrot, the preacher is searching for salvation, patients are looking for quality health care, states are looking for lower health care costs, and practitioners want stability and less interference in their practice. In the end, only the rabbit will be happy.

Chapter Two

Private Practice Is Not Private

The previous chapter addressed the transition of health care services from a cottage industry to a health care industry within the context of the administrative posture of managed care. With this transition has come an increase in stature for corporations contracting with state and federal agencies. They have attained political power and financial assets. The capital has come from Wall Street; the political power from lobbyists and Congress. The business side of health care has sprung out of managed care's tentacles of influence in the political and business arenas. As health care researchers, theorists, and writers have explored the influence of suggestion, of various therapies, and of new medications, managed care has used its position to reign in both the positive side of health care services as well as the negative, or those who deliberately attempt to create schemes that focus on building pots of gold rather than helping patients overcome disease, disorders, disparity, and despair.

It is not surprising that the demand for health care services has been rising. There have been new technologies, new medications, and improved techniques to address chronic pain, loss of limbs and mobility, and dissatisfaction with daily life activities. Generally speaking, people prefer life to death and a feeling of inner balance rather than turmoil and pain. Therapies that add years of quality to a life or that allow a person to participate in daily life events and activities are now in greater demand. The business community understands how demand increases sales, but in health care an increase in demand is unwelcome due to the increased exposure to additional costs, both short and long-term. Therefore, every effort is made legislatively with Wall Street corporations to tighten the control over health care products, services, and providers. Control may also mean that corporations are formed to take over a new procedure or technology and then they participate at both ends of health care: administrative and delivery. For example, pharmacy benefit managers (PBMs), who are third party administrators, advertise that people have a choice as to where they fill their prescriptions. These managers are primarily responsible for processing and paying prescription drug claims. They also can develop and maintain a drug formulary, which is a list of medications normally used by different health care plans including Medicare, Medicaid, and the Federal Employees Health Benefit Program. The managers contract with pharmacies, negotiating discounts and rebates with drug manufacturers in order to save the consumer money, but also to attract more consumers and physicians to their program. It has been suggested that more than 200 million Americans nationwide receive drug benefits administered by a PBM. PBMs have been a resource for many people; however, when one or more of these corporations decide to limit choices to a single pharmacy chain, which they own, problems develop for the consumer. One such plan changed their policy and their customers received correspondence that stated, "You will pay the entire cost of these prescriptions if you continue to fill those long-term prescriptions at a retail pharmacy." Then the letter offered to fill their prescriptions "and your prescriptions will be sent right to you, with free shipping for standard delivery" (Lazarus, 2012, pp. 1-2). One consumer complained that he has been with his pharmacist for 30 years and now Medco is saying that he can only buy from them. Such actions, which increase profit margins for Medco, are putting many pharmacies out of business. A small mom-and-pop pharmacy, which used to be considered a private practice, is no longer private and now takeovers by managed care or PBMs are making family pharmacies obsolete.

Big Brother is alive and more active than George Orwell ever dreamed possible. If sales are paid for, at least in part, by insurance companies, Medicaid, or Medicare, there are costs involved with the acceptance of these plans. This does not equate with the individual services or medicines automatically increasing. Providers that exhibit a certain naiveté about the effects of this demand on the practice of health care have been hindered in seeing the waves of change hitting the shore, impacting the structure of the health care environment and the playing field. Corporate America is acting foolishly since they are the ones who invented marketing, as well as the ones who created ways to monitor unit costs. They are purposely contributing misinformation so that premiums will go down on their employees' health benefits package. They in turn raise the rates of the products they are involved with, such as gasoline, clothing, interest rates on loans and credit cards, transportation costs, and many more. The economic theory of tension that moves the direction of supply and demand has also impacted the price of the unit of production or service.

Within the discussions of health care reform come questions about expansions in the debt or expense column without a reciprocal credit to the revenue column. As noted above, health care services are offering what patients want and, as any marketing representative knows, greater demand means higher sales and increased profits for the manufacturers. In the auto industry General Motors has departments that are created to promote sales and others to protect the product against legislation that restricts their ability to trade in the open marketplace. They also have lobbyists vociferating to Congress for protection from rising insurance premiums that are adding to the costs per unit. Each dollar that is added on translates into $100 of income lost to a competitor. We might hear words such as socialism and entitlements that are replaced by democratic entrepreneurships. Strange as it sounds, General Motors of America is encouraged and helped during financial downswings and then applauded during years of profit, whereas health care providers are said to be greedy and more interested in padding their bank accounts than in providing services. There are no two General Motors and no two providers that look alike; however, that does not stop people from making generalities which are demeaning. Using words to demean or reward are ways of separating one from another by intimidation or by building up support, which is similar to the efforts of one group trying to control another group. In this case, the population in the highest level of social economic development is attempting to protect their billions of dollars in investments and savings at the expense of the lower social economic group.

Corporations blame increased product costs on the rising health care premiums that they must pass on to the consumer. For example, when consumers see less expensive automobiles from Japan or Germany; they see that they have a choice. Car manufacturers argue that they need Congress to cut the rising premiums to their corporations. Congress has offered bailouts for the car industry, the banking industry, and Wall Street corporations. The bailout money pays the costs of changing their products in order to become more competitive, but it also pays their top management millions of dollars in yearly bonuses. There has been no talk about bailing out the health care industry. Instead the talk is about curbing health care production. Congress has authorized a greater number of law enforcement entities and managed care companies to join forces in order to take control of hospitals and health care providers. More audit providers have been added to law enforcement and managed care organizations. In addition laws allowing for greater interest rates for the recoupment program have been enacted, and in order to monitor provider offices and billing practices, case management has been expanded. Such a message tells the consumer that the providers are the ones increasing the costs of health care; that they are to blame for the loss of mental health services, dental services, or speech therapy services. Such messages, whether expressed or inferred, interfere with the relationship of provider and patient. This interference comes in the form of creating doubt in the patient's mind about the quality of care while fearing the loss of their

health care provider. Patients do not understand the positioning struggle between their provider and the HMO; knowledge and desire for a health care
service, both medical and mental health, is paramount to the patient regardless of the politics of health care administration, financing, and delivery
(Brezosky, 2012, p. 19).

A long-time problem facing providers are the issues that have made them
become like sheep, acting as if nothing is ever going to make them change
their practice. This type of thinking has delayed physicians and allied providers from accepting the business side of health care and in learning how and
why it is suddenly shaking and re-shaping their practice. "The single biggest
issue for the providers is that they don't know what their internal production
costs are and have no knowledge of their external production costs" (Burns,
2012, p. 43). As private practices are being closed, providers find that they
have choices, although not all of them are lucrative. Now providers are
learning to adjust, as they have been suggesting to their patients for years.
They are setting new priorities, paying off debts, selling assets that have no
future utility, and they are taking their many years of experience with them.

Over the years providers have made many mistakes: they have lost their
business savvy, have not wanted to see their profession as part of the health
care industry, and have avoided sharing what they have learned with new
graduates in their field. In addition they have not been active enough in
standing up for their value to society (Cummings and O'Donohue, 2008).
The cost of health care is not too high when it comes to VALUE, such as
saving a life, helping a paralyzed person to walk again, and mending broken
hearts and spirits (Burns, 2002; Callahan, 2003; Cutler, 2004).

THE BATTLE FOR POWER

Power is the opium of management, whether it's government or large corporations. The battle for power over the health care industry is fought by:

- Federal Government
- State Government
- Wall Street Corporations
- A loose group of providers, professional organizations, patients, and pa-
  tient's rights groups

The first group is composed of politicians, federal layers of departments, and
divisions of bureaucracy. The second group is composed of state governments with their layers of departments and divisions of bureaucracy. The
third group is composed of corporations that trade on the New York Stock
Exchange, including lobbyists, banking corporations, and pharmaceutical in-

dustries. The last group is made up of unions, professional associations, providers, patients, and patient's rights groups and activists. The last group has little significance other than the role they play to help the other groups achieve their goals.

The third group contributes funding for many of the hospital chains across the nation. They have also had a hand in the manufacturing of medications that have helped to relieve and control pain, and they are active supporters of the first two groups because they benefit the most from what the first two groups plan, including legislative regulations. The lobbyists are the surrogates for the corporations who funnel finances to Super Pacs and to legislators who support their causes. The first two groups need this group to generate expertise in finances and economic issues, such as projections and theories; in management, in the development or reconstructions of organizational structures; in banking, to offer the best ways to finance projects and control revenue sources; and in law enforcement, to develop the best forensic examiners for information gathering, audit analyses, prediction of fraud abuse, and prosecution assistance in case development in prosecuting fraud cases.

THE POWER OF MONEY

The struggle over power and money has led to an inability to protect the clinical field of practice from those whose corporate goals are to make money, not for the industry, but for themselves. The influence of money runs towards other sources, such as competition in the profession, in the marketplace, and in government. Political influence feeds on anything that increases profit margins. The larger the profit margin, the more attractive the product or service becomes. Big corporations have used leverage techniques to buy out positioning power at the legislative table where government programs are created and opportunities for contract work are manufactured. The chief executive officer, CEO, is the highest executive officer in a corporation and is the one who answers to the board of directors. The CEO is the dreamer, the global thinker, the one making the most difficult decisions for the corporation that point to commitment of revenues and resources for the future. The chief financial officer, CFO, is the highest financial officer in a corporation and is the one who presents the corporate budget and financial instruments to the CEO. Chief operating officers, COOs, are the top three officer positions behind the CEO and CFO, and they have the responsibility of day-to-day operations. Health care providers are not acquainted with these acronyms; they are more acquainted with their title as granted by their licensing board, or their degree, or administrative authority. As the transition from a cottage industry into a giant health care industry has taken place, the need has risen for more expertise in managing practices. Therefore, in the past 20 years new administrative jobs have been born due to various needs:

- Statistical analysis,
- Detection of inappropriate billing
- Discovering acts of health care or health insurance fraud
- Developing case managers and other administrators within the managed care organization to monitor populations of billing trends and patient file documentation.

Managed care organizations have developed an expertise in risk management, loss containment, and risk and liability control.

One of the reasons these three groups of corporate leadership make so much money is that they know how to predict trends and how to form departments and programs for change before talk of change even begins. When the Obama Act of 2010 was signed into law, corporate boards were deliberating and lower level management was having committee meetings while reading the regulations, as well as all the material from the Department of Health and Human Services, analyzing how insurance carriers and administrators would be impacted. They know what to expect before the information is supplied to the media who, in turn, write articles in their blogs and newspapers to share this information with providers and patients. The push for creating interdisciplinary collaborations is growing. Mental and physical health parity in Oregon's Blue Cross Blue Shield subsidiary, Regency, announced they are cutting out mental health services and raising deductibles for individual and small group policies. They can do this because they are a corporation whose mission is to make money for their stockholders. They can do this because the federal government rules for parity begins with a group of 50 and above, thus the loophole has once again saved the day for corporate America. For psychologists and psychiatrists who are building cash only practices, this can be helpful. For those depending on insurance reimbursements, it can be very painful.

In managing businesses, financial officers and bankers use profit and loss (P&Ls) statements as a way of determining financial strength. Included within the P&Ls are a balance sheet, a cash flow statement, and an income statement. P&Ls summarize the revenues as well as the costs and expenses incurred during a specific period of time, normally each quarter. A balance sheet is a quick look at the financial position of a company at any given point in time. An income statement addresses the amount of revenue generated and the expenses incurred over a period of time, normally a quarter. Return on investments (ROIs) is a term that describes the process of accounting for the rate or amount received on investments over a period of time. Bankers and investment counselors work with ROIs daily, as do many certified public accountants (CPAs). ROI is a measure of a corporation's profitability. Accounting formulas and techniques are used to measure how effectively a business uses its capital to generate profit; the idea is to increase the ROIs so that a company becomes more profitable and financially stable.

ROIs have been discussed here because we, as providers, need to be more conscious of the value of making a profit. Profit is not a bad word. Providers should become aware of ways to use the ROIs for their practices and also for personal family benefits, up to and including retirement years; however, it may mean that we find another occupation since profit, in a health care context, is a nasty word. Now even WORDS are being controlled for the health care industry. While hospitals seem to be immune to the term, primary care physicians, mental health specialists, physical therapists, chiropractors, and others find it distasteful because they are still operating in a cottage industry mentality, supported by the attitudes of patients and government agencies.

The Department of Defense has learned quickly when it comes to creating different sources of power for the war effort that could be financed in a way not revealed on their defense budgets, where Congress reviews and then approves or questions. They have created a second army that goes into battle as support and a resource for commanders without increasing the number of military members in the field. Thousands of military lives were lost in WWI and WWII; since then, the lives lost in Vietnam, Iraq, and Afghanistan have been minimal in comparison. This is due in part to new techniques for battle that allow troops to stay further away from the enemy while attacking with weapons that can reach the enemy hundreds of miles away. Advances in triage and treatment of patients closer to the battlefield have also saved lives. Wars are normally managed by military commanders and high ranking officers. They have the duty to report and collaborate with the Secretaries of the Army, Navy, Marines, Air Force, and the Coast Guard and whose highest ranking officer reports to the Secretary of Defense who, in turn, reports to the President of the United States, to the President's Cabinet, and to Congress.

The war effort in Iraq and in the Middle Eastern countries over the last ten years can be used as an example of how military missions are receiving help on the battlefield from Wall Street corporations. The contracts for services in support of the war effort have made small corporations large and big corporation giants of their industry. Such is the case with the following corporations as reported from Pentagon records:

- KBR/Halliburton ($2.329 billion)
- Bechtel ($1.030 billion)
- International American Products ($527 million)
- Perini Corporation ($525 million)
- Contract International ($500 million)

- Fluor ($500 million)
- Washington Group International ($500 million)
- Research Triangle Institute ($466 million)
- Louis Berger Group ($300 million)
- Creative Associates International ($217 million) (Beelman, 2003)

In the history of war there is no comparison as to the ways contractors have been used to support various military efforts. The contractors have been in almost every area of action, from where the military was holding maneuvers or developing strategies for controlling the region, to even in the Green Zone of Baghdad, Iraq. People from Africa were hired as security guards and positioned on the walls around the Green Zone; others were hired to be body guards for members of Congress, at UFO events, and some were even used as counselors, computer technicians, weapon designers, and manufacturers. There have been as many contractors in the war zone as there have been soldiers and airmen, but we haven't adjusted our thinking because of this. We haven't adjusted our structure for it either, reported Charles Tiefer, member of the Commission on Wartime Contracting and a professor of government contracting at the University of Baltimore Law School (Goodman & Gonzalez, 2011).

> One such company was Tucson-based Applied Energetics, which markets a futuristic weapon that shoots beams of lightning to detonate roadside bombs. The company won over $50 million in military contracts for their lightning weapon; all without full and open competition, even though there was another company marketing a similar technology. Despite test failures, the company, in part because of congressional support, continued to get funding (Weinberger, 2011).

THE INFLUENCE OF COSTS

During the past 15 years more attention has been given to the business side of health care practices, largely from the debate over health care costs. Patients have died because they could not afford treatment or medications. Non-profit hospitals and clinics have tried to fill the gap, but there are still over 43 million Americans that are either uninsured or underinsured. Debate has focused on costs to state and national budgets. Governors are cutting programs to try to balance the budget through slashing services because the alternative, raising taxes, is political suicide. Therefore, whenever a program is discussed that affects health care services, political and corporate groups bring in illuminating sound bites such as: it's another entitlement program; that bill promotes socialism; if we have a national health insurance bill then we will have a worse problem with immigration.

In spite of these arguments President Obama offered what he saw as a compromise program: the Patient Protection and Affordable Care Act of 2010. The Act was first defeated in 2009 and was one of three legislative bills, which included a single provider universal health care program that was defeated. A revised legislative bill was signed into law in March of 2010, which was a compromise among political adversaries. The passed bills are now known as the Patient Protection and Affordable Care Act, as well as the Health Care and Education Reconciliation Act. Many of the provisions have a timeline that extends to 2014. The primary goal of this Act is to create a program to include most of those that are now uninsured or underinsured. This translates into millions of people who will now be eligible to purchase a health care policy even though they have cancer, diabetes, or degenerative heart failure.

There is also the issue of insurance and practice fraud. With the Act, efforts have been made to collaborate with other federal and state agents to combat what is expected to be a greater problem with fraudulent claims in 2014 when millions are brought into the Medicaid programs. An article published by Health Affairs addressed these concerns:

> CMS's estimate of improper payments, which relies on random samples of claims data, is widely thought to understate the true size of the problem of fraud and abuse. In an April 2012 study, former CMS administrator Donald M. Berwick and RAND Corporation analyst Andrew D. Hackbarth estimated that fraud and abuse added as much as $98 billion to Medicare and Medicaid spending in 2011.

> For many years, the Government Accountability Office (GAO), the investigative arm of Congress, has designated Medicare and Medicaid as being at "high risk" for fraud, abuse, and improper payments. Both programs were designed to enroll "any willing provider" and to reimburse claims quickly for services provided.

> Although CMS is optimistic about the potential of these new techniques, many consider the results thus far to be disappointing. As of January 6, 2012, only $7,591 in payments had been suspended as a consequence of use of advanced analytics. CMS officials have acknowledged a lag time between discovering violations and reporting them in public documents. But they also point out that every line in each of Medicare's daily 4.5 million fee-for-service claims is now examined through some form of analytics, and that new analytical models are introduced each quarter, which should lead to better results from use of this antifraud technology over time (Health Affairs, 2012, pp. 1-5).

Fraudulent claims increase the cost of doing business for the HMOs, MCOs, and the state and federal governments. It is a realistic concern and those who commit fraud should be punished. Unfortunately, state agencies can become overzealous when they attack health care programs and organizations that have been "too successful." One therapist developed a mental health organization in San Antonio, Texas, and after several years they came after him with a three-year investigation, at the end of which they gave him back all his files without stating any allegations to him or to his attorney. The agents involved claimed that he was the target of the investigation in which the IRS, FBI, Inspector General, and the Attorney General's office attempted to prove money laundering and insurance fraud. "You were just too big," they offered. In most industries people are honored and respected for making a successful business or product, but in health care that is only done with mega hospital organizations.

RECOUPMENT

For health care providers the term recoupment is foreign, for banks and insurance companies, it is fairly common, and for the Department of Health and Human Services, it is not new. In one publication an example is given of how the recoupment rate is determined in a welfare program:

> Ms. A and her child live in a Group II county. Mr. A receives child support of $100 per month for the child included in the GA family unit. She and her child receive a GA benefit of $207 ($307 payment level minus $100 countable income). She has an outstanding overpayment of $300.

To determine the amount that can be recouped from her monthly GA benefit:

- Her level of income cannot be reduced more than 90% of her Payment Level: $307 x 90% = $276.30.
- Her income without the GA benefit = $100.
- Her GA benefit must bring her level of income to $276.30; $276.30 minus $100 = $176.30.
- The amount that can be recouped = $207 minus $176.30 = $30.70.

Example 2: A mother, father, and their 2 children receive GA benefits. An overpayment is established against the GA case. The father leaves the home. Recoupment continues, as the mother was part of the original overpaid GA case (DHHS, 2012).

The Centers for Medicare & Medicaid Services, CMS, has been using recoupment for quite some time, and many vendors are accustomed to their demand letters. Providers, on the other hand, are normally unaware of what recoupment means and how it works. When the OSG sends out a letter they do not explain about the interest rate or how they determine why recoupment is necessary. Those in private practice, who accept Medicaid, are ill prepared for recoupment and see it as another way to reduce reimbursements and to add expenses to the budget of the provider without recourse. Here is what appeared in a February 10, 2012 newsletter:

> Effective July 1, 2012, however, providers can request recoupment to begin prior to day 41. Providers who elect this process may avoid the assessment of interest if the overpayment is paid back in full before day 31. Providers who voluntarily choose immediate recoupment must do so in writing (by mail, FAX, or email) to contractors. The letter should contain the following information:
>
> • Provider name and phone number
> • Provider Medicare number and/or National Provider Identifier (NPI)
> • Provider or CFO's signature
> • Demand letter number
> • Which option the provider is requesting

Providers can elect a one-time immediate recoupment request for the current overpayment and all future overpayments or request immediate recoupment for a specific overpayment addressed in a demand letter. A request for an immediate recoupment letter must be received by contractors no later than the 16th day from the date of the initial demand letter.

> In accordance with 42 CFR 405.378, simple interest at the rate of 10.50 percent (effective Jan. 19, 2012) will be charged on the unpaid balance of the overpayment beginning on the 31st day. Interest is calculated in 30-day periods and is assessed for each full 30-day period that payment is not made on time. In other words, if payment is received 31 days from the date of final determination, one 30-day period of interest will be charged (AAPC, 2012).

The OSG sends letters out about recoupment and will address the issue of appeal in the letter but the appeal process differs from state to state. For example, New Jersey law states there must be 45 days for notice of recoupment, that the state can go back 18 months of claims, and that: the payer may only seek reimbursement once; payer must provide written documentation of error and justification; provider may appeal within 45 days; if no appeal payer can attach future claims, but payer must give sufficient detail to allow account reconciliation (Medical Society of New Jersey, 2012).

In the state of Texas an appeal is not allowed until the entire amount is paid off, and there is a limited period of time in which to appeal. Those who have no experience with this type of program or with the process of appeal would do well to consult with a legal firm who specializes in such cases. While it is unlikely that they will be able to eliminate the entire amount, they may save the provider money if they can determine if the justification for recoupment is faulty. Recoupment is becoming more widespread. It is becoming common practice to have a letter sent from an insurance carrier announcing to the administrators that one of their tasks is recoupment. Administrators offer different formulas for recoupment: Aetna and Cigna offer 30 days' notice of recoupment; Healthnet offers 90 days; Aetna will go back two years for recoupment; Cigna and Healthnet only 12 months; Aetna and Cigna offer 30 days to file a compliance dispute while Healthnet offers 90 days for such action. The process of filing a dispute claim with OSG, as well as understanding the appeal process and the arbitration process, are issues of which few medical personnel have any knowledge. There are attorneys in most state capitals, as well as major metropolitan communities that specialize in such actions; however, prepare to pay a substantial sum for their services. If a recoupment amount is less than $10,000, spending another $10,000 for a legal team may not be wise. The other issue is the legal system that supports the state is so stacked against individual health care providers of any discipline and license that they can appeal all the way to the Department of Health and Human Services, and it could be a waste of time, energy, and money.

One of their assigned tasks is to run a recoupment program for the state run Medicaid program. This term is not familiar to most providers and is becoming a thorn in their sides. For the past two years the Solicitor General's office in Texas, and perhaps in other states, has started a campaign to recover money paid to providers through a system that is more common in the banking and insurance industry than in health care. For health care providers recoupment means the practice of claiming money from past reimbursements out of future claim payments. The state justifies this collection process due to a belief that there have been over payments made, and through a conflated rationale that is as confusing as most legal documents, leaves more questions than answers. This agency is filled with lawyers, accountants, law enforcement administrators, and attorneys that may explain the language problem.

The Solicitor General's office, within the state's Medicaid administration, serves as another law enforcement agency embedded into a federal or state program. Their job is to gather data to assimilate into potential legal cases against health care providers who may see more patients each year than the norm for their license or for the codes used for billing. Such scenarios are red flags that attract closer surveillance. Their assumption is that providers who bill fee-for-services are tempted to increase their billings at the risk of inappropriate billing, or even insurance fraud. In Texas, the Solicitor General's office has focused on curtailing or stopping family therapy billings. They do this by targeting clinics that may be billing more for family services than others of similar licenses. The fact that clinics organized to meet the needs of family services and excel at helping families learn better parenting skills, how to reduce family violence, and help to increase school attendance and thus better grades for their children, does not seem to faze their stoic and narrow vision. There are a number of mental health issues that are presented at such sessions and include children with ADD/ADHD, excessive aggression, depression, anxiety, poor self-regulation of anger, and oppositional defiance that disrupts family life as well as school successes, both behavioral and academic.

The Solicitor General only knows statistics and ignores the additional information that could explain a rise in family sessions. The agency also ignores the fact that statistics can be used to explain any position the Solicitor General wishes to take. In addition, when an audit is performed, a list providing dates of services is presented to the therapist along with a request for copies of the progress notes of predetermined dates. Within six weeks they return a demand for reimbursement of thousands of dollars, which they claim the therapist is estimated to owe them for overbilling. When challenged, they can send another registered letter demanding more money and claiming the time of service, diagnostic codes, proof of the need for family services, inadequate note taking, and illegible notes were not listed. There is an appeal process, but that cannot be initiated until all the funds have been paid. There is no hearing, no explanation of proof beyond vague claims, and references to various bulletins found on the Medicaid website. These bulletins read like legal forms and legislative bills that are easily misunderstood by both providers and law enforcement personnel in the Medicaid administration.

To challenge the allegations with the assistance of a legal team will cost at least $10,000 and can go even higher as the process is extended. One owner of a group practice was charged $250,000 due to the fact that one of her psychologists signed her progress notes with initials. The owner of this group practice fought it for several years, but eventually she lost both her business and her practice. Others have practiced 30 years or more and have gone through inspections, but have never experienced the mean-spirited attitude that is now being presented. While not everyone is this difficult to communicate with, in order to make any headway through the maze of bureaucratic defense posturing without legal representation is next to impossible. The Solicitor General's use of administrative and judicial influence can apply leverage techniques to run private practitioners out of business; one podiatrist was asked for $345,000! Governor Perry's rationale for deep cuts in Medicaid programs is due to the fact that Texas faces a $3.9 billion deficit in the Texas Medicaid obligation for next year. According to Perry the cost of Medicaid is a ticking time bomb and is primed to do major damage to our budget in both the short and long terms. (Fikac, 2012, p.A6). Texas has one of the highest rates of uninsured individuals in the nation. The need for these services is there, the demand is growing, but the Governor of Texas says no and, as a result, patients lose. While Governor Perry can argue that a blue ribbon committee made the decision, the committee was selected by Mr. Perry and his staff. When the committee is asked for an explanation, they blame the Department of Health and Human Services. The buck never stops on any one desk; it keeps being pushed around until the questioner goes away or dies. Government always has more time and resources than do patients and providers.

"The fact is, in most medical practices the margin is so low, that to take away 20%, puts the patient in a situation where it costs the provider more in office expenses to see the patient," states Dr. Bruce Malone, president of the Texas Medical Association. "There's no business in the world that can function that way" (Brezosky, 2012, p. 19). If non-health care corporations were made to operate in the same environment and with similar legislation, there would be a drastic shutdown of NAFTA trade, and other trade agreements would not be worth the paper they were written on, as corporations would begin drastically cutting back or closing.

AFFORDABLE CARE ORGANIZATIONS

The Affordable Care Act of 2010 includes a section on the development of Affordable Care Organizations, ACOs. This affects health care providers of all disciplines, as it is an attempt by the federal government to force the coordination of information and services within the health care industry. One of the goals of ACOs is to encourage local control over the growth of health care spending and also to encourage the improvement of quality over quantity of care. Each ACO performance will be monitored on a number of quality measures that are expected to ensure that the organization is accessing mental health, in addition to hospitals and primary care services. Performance benefits are offered to encourage reaching quality goals.

The following is a brief summary of the Act and the years certain parts were implemented:

2010

- Young adults that are working but are not covered under their employer's health care plan can be covered under their parents' plan until they turn 26.
- Some preventive care services are made mandatory without a deductible.
- Insurance companies are now prohibited from imposing lifetime dollar amounts to health coverage.
- Children under 19 years of age cannot be denied health coverage due to a pre-existing condition.

2011

- Senior citizens who reach the prescription-coverage gap associated with Medicare Part D brand-name prescriptions receive a 50% discount of future purchases of prescription medications.
- All Medicare recipients receive free preventative care.
- Insurance companies are forced to spend 85% of all premium dollars on health care services under several conditions.

2012

- Incentives for physicians to form Accountable Care Organizations, which is a way of forcing collaboration with other providers (medical and allied professionals, such as psychologists, chiropractors, physical therapists, substance abuse counselors, and psychotherapists).
- A voluntary long-term care insurance program was created.
- Medical paperwork begins to be converted to electronic files.
- A value-based purchasing program was established.

2013

- Medicaid funding programs begin to offer preventive care services with little to no cost to patients.
- Federal funds are released to reimburse primary care providers of Medicare & Medicaid patients at 100% of Medicare rates. Most primary physicians lost the co-payment on the Medicaid coverage in 2010.
- Insurance coverage for children not eligible for Medicaid is extended by two years.

2014

- All pre-existing medical conditions are eliminated.
- If employers do not offer insurance, employees can purchase a policy through their state exchange program.
- All Americans who earn less than 133% of the poverty level receive a Medicaid policy.
- Annual limits on insurance coverage are eliminated.
- Business tax credits up to 50% of the employer-paid portion of an employee's health insurance premiums are allowed (Withrow, 2012, pp. 1-3).

The Act of 2010 has implications that go further than what this book has room to explain even if every nuance was understood. The problem with legislative action is that legislators do not read ahead of time the things on which they vote. Then there is the issue of legislative bills having their own jargon, their own acronyms, and they often need a group of attorneys to explain. For example, the Act is a long bill and public officials have been candid with their admission of not reading it first. The same thing happens in state legislatures. In Texas, in 2009, a bill was passed that included a section cutting billable hours that mental health providers could bill for a family therapy session per day. While that might seem reasonable at face value, there are clinical issues that can occur that require more than an hour of therapy. No provision for exceptions was made, and the confusion over how to apply this ruling has led to the Solicitor General asking for reimbursement from over 500 providers who had no knowledge of this bill. When their legislators were contacted, they remember the bill but not that particular section. Everyone wants to save money, but the bill was unclear and other sections distracted from this one application and its possible consequences (therapists having to pay back thousands of dollars). Also the provision stated that therapists, or social workers, could not appeal the process until they had paid the money back. This rationale is in direct conflict with the judicial agencies that do not require a death penalty, or any prison term, to be completed before the appeal process can begin.

The Centers for Medicare & Medicaid Services (ACA) received over 1300 letters addressing the weaknesses of the ACO regulations and refusing to participate as an ACO. Their comments included:

- The requirement of ACOs to pay back CMS funds if the ACO ended up speeding the growth in their health care spending instead of slowing it down (in other words, communities that expand populations could easily see an increase in services, not because they performed poorly but due to the fact that there were more patients seeking medical and mental health needs than prior to the ACO's formation)
- Not counting specialists' patients in ACOs
- Tie bonuses to performances on 65 quality measures
- Requiring 50 percent of an ACO's primary care physicians to be meaningful users of electronic health records (Berenson and Burton, 2011, pp. 1-3)

These arguments were reviewed by CMS and some changes were made. While demonstrations of selected ACO experiments suggest that quality of care can be improved, the jury is out about the amount of savings that can be expected. The bottom line in support of this type of experiment is how spending can be curtailed with significant numbers.

COORDINATED CARE ORGANIZATIONS

Not all states have bought into the ACO program and instead have developed their own programs for encouraging providers to collaborate. Oregon's program is called the Coordinated Care Organization Implementation Proposal (House Bill 3650, Health Care Transformation, January 10, 2012.) According to this bill the four essential elements of this program are:

- Integration and coordination of benefits and services
- Local accountability for health and resource allocation
- Standards for safe and effective care
- A global Medicaid budget tied to a sustainable rate of growth (Oregon, 2012, p. 1)

Like the ACO program, Oregon's legislature wants a community-based organization governed by a partnership between providers of care, community members, and those taking financial risk. While Oregon acknowledges that the current system has been able to offer quality services, there is a question that the current structure of services has its limits and that there is value in integrating and coordinating patient-centered health care services. Oregon also endorses the need to curb costs. The new proposal supports increased efficiency, recognition of value of health care, prevention strategies, and wellness outcomes. Like the ACOs there is a built-in system for accountability.

The American Mental Health Alliance, AMHA, with their Oregon chapter, has offered another term to reach similar goals: Connecting Care. This organization has been very active in helping their members to be prepared for the health care reform movements in member states. They champion patients' rights, confidentiality, and professionalism of their members. Their program members have a website that elucidates the principle issues of the organization and also presents pictures and information about each member's practice. Connecting Care's goals are:

- To improve the health of the population
- To enhance the patient experience, which includes quality, access, and reliability
- To manage, or contain, the per capita cost of care (Mentor Research Institute, 2012, p.1)

This model has seven primary functions:

- A referral system that connects physicians and patients with qualified and appropriate counselors, social workers, and psychologists

- Evidence-based measurement of referral effectiveness, including progress and outcomes
- Practice management, including billing, electronic health records, and auditing data between physicians and mental health professionals
- Clinic and community based screenings
- Risk assessment screening that supports public safety
- A health education resource that includes written content and videos (Mentor Research Institute, 2012, p. 1)

There are many possibilities that seem to be on the horizon in regards to Congress and the White House; however, leaders of reform have not done enough to understand the needs of providers, including primary care physicians. Medical doctors are concerned about losses in reimbursement rates, which have already been cut to those with mental health licenses. Secondly, doctors were told that Medicare reimbursement rates would not be cut until 2013, but Medicaid is now refusing to pay for co-payments on Medicare-Medicaid coverage, which translates into discounted reimbursement. Such political double talk is similar to what happened 25 years ago with the advent of managed care panels. Physicians were encouraged to join hospital panels, but after a short period of time many were dismissed after they challenged the decisions of the managed care auditors or gatekeepers. One of the issues of reimbursement rates for any health care discipline begins with the discussion of value. The Centers for Medicare and Medicaid Services (CMS) has the responsibility to address this issue; beginning with how much time and effort is associated with various services. The CMS must rely on the recommendations of advisory committees who represent national physicians and services from the fields of mental health, physical therapy, chiropractic, and speech therapy. At stake is the discrepancy between primary care physicians and specialists in the medical field, who are blamed for the shortage of primary care physicians.

PHARMACEUTICAL INDUSTRY

Pharmacies are hit hard, too, with the cuts in health care reform. In the state of Texas Medicaid reimbursement rates have been reduced from $6.50 to $1.35 for dispensing fees for each prescription, which is below cost. In many parts of Texas, especially rural and border communities, there are many low income populations who are covered by Medicaid. With the population of those who will be covered by Medicaid increasing over the next four years, this will mean that pharmacies will need to add additional personnel. When the dispersing rate per unit of cost is below the cost line, the company will lose not only their normal profit, but it will cost them more to operate. This means that they could work themselves out of business. Budgets that are in the black are making a profit and those in the red are losing money.

"My prediction is that we'll lose 20 percent of the pharmacies in the rural areas within six months," stated Marv Shepherd, director of the Center for Pharmacoeconomic Studies at the University of Texas at Austin. People are going to have to drive 50 miles to find a pharmacy that accepts Medicaid. An industry-funded study by the Perryman Group estimated the cuts would put 1,300 Texas pharmacies in the red. (Finley, 2012, p. B3).

SUPER PACS

Pharmacies and mental health providers are taking huge deficits to help stabilize state budgets; doctors, nurses, nursing homes, home health services, and hospitals, as well as other allied providers, can expect to get hit hard too. The only ones not affected are the state and federal legislators, governors, Supreme Court justices, and the President of the United States. Other groups that are not losing money are the lobbyists and political action committees, PACs.

> "It's not about (political) party it's about process," stated Curtis Ellis, a Houston spokesman for the Campaign for Primary Accountability. "We want the people of Congress to fear Main Street, not K Street. Super PACs can raise money and receive unlimited amounts from donors, but they are not allowed to coordinate directly with candidates or political parties" (Martin, 2012).

Main Street is normally used to refer to the common man. There is nothing common about the Super PACs and no common man has enough money to donate to these organizations. The PACs are about political power and they have the money to leverage any deal they choose. Super PACs are formed to raise money to spend in media advertisements either advocating a position for one candidate, or using a negative advertisement to distract from a candidate or issue. Unlike formal campaigns, there are no contribution limits and they are subjected to different Federal Election Commission reporting requirements. They are restricted from coordinating with any campaign, and there are no requirements to identify donors or to disclose where the money originated. There is a limit on how much a Super Pac can donate to a candidate in each election ($2,500).

NATIONALISM AND/OR SOCIALISM

During the 2012 presidential election Mitt Romney threw out the term "socialism" as if it were a dirty word. His comments surround the "entitlement programs" where he claimed 47% of Americans withdraw retirement dollars, disability, or some social welfare program dollars out of the national/state budgets. He also suggested that this 47% does not vote, or at least a majority do not vote, at any election. Romney wanted to see the entitlement program cut by some percentage to help reduce the national and state budgets. Social welfare programs have a long history in America as Americans are normally for the underdog, and as such, frequently contribute to Goodwill, veteran programs, and the American Red Cross. When disasters hit a part of the country, Americans have volunteered money, time, energy, resources, supplies, and food for people hurt by the disaster. Most providers of health care enter the profession because they like to help others. America has been very conscious of the religious principles that contributed to the birth of America and the framing of the U.S. Constitution. One of the creeds that has been promoted throughout our history is the biblical statute: Do unto others as you would have done to you (Luke 6:31).

There is another side to socialism that the current generation may not understand or appreciate. Some countries have communistic policies that encompass socialistic programs of dividing goods and supplies to families, which often results in huge lines like America had during the great depression when people stood in line for bread and other grocery items. Before the Berlin Wall came down, East Germany and other countries next to them were "trained" by standing daily in bread lines. When they could travel to West Germany, they were embraced with money and offered a job; however, as my West German friends reported, they did not know how to work, so most returned to East Germany earlier rather than later.

Socialism has its dark side in that there is no private practice in a socialistic government-run country. Again from Merriam-Webster dictionary, under a socialistic government the production is controlled by the government. There is a transitional point between communism and capitalism, where there is "unequal distribution of goods and pay according to work done." One certainly can argue that we have some programs that may sound socialistic and that capitalism is similar to the elitists that run a socialistic government.

Nationalism refers to the government controlling an industry, having a dominate rule of order, and dictating to citizens through the federal law enforcement, as well as state and county law enforcement and judicial systems. Merriam-Webster Dictionary says that nationalism is showing pride in your country and exalting your country over all others. This sounds like most Americans today as we will stand when the flag goes by, or salute the flag, and we sing the national anthem at different events. At the Olympics we often yell cries of "USA, USA, USA"; however, people tend to cringe when they hear that the federal government is going to take over an industry such as the railroads, bus transportation, or the post office. This is different than giving the industry or organization a loan with an interest rate to help "bail out a floundering corporation so that thousands of employees can keep their jobs.

It can also refer to the managing of a budget problem, such as when President Obama introduced his health care program. The oppositional party called it socialism, which can be another word for nationalization. This means the government takes control of an industry. Congress authorized states to hire organizations to act as surrogates who have the power to take over the state Medicaid health care administration (MCOs and HMOs, and special law enforcement agencies searching for fraud, money laundering, and over billing). When government takes over the banks within their national boundaries, it is called nationalizing the banking industry. The government claims that they are doing it to protect the interests of the nation and those who have money in the banks. Nationalization has also been used when there is an acquisition by legal maneuvering that allows a company to petition the state to pronounce a portion of land, which is owned by others, as eminent domain. One way this is done is to purchase water or mineral rights on a ranch and then, through eminent domain, force their way onto the land to dig across the ranch in order to place large pipes that will carry oil or natural gas from Canada to South Texas to be processed in another corporation's refinery. People in South Texas have talked about corporations offering to buy the mineral rights, including water rights, of ranchers. There has been media coverage of how cities, or states, have taken private property for public purposes such as the construction of roads, dams, or public buildings. They do it as a right of eminent domain. The dark side of nationalism is the program of eminent domain which means the state can use it to cut dirt out of your ranch and sell the space to a foreign government to run gas through the pipes. Or taking over one's house, giving them some money, and then tearing the house down to build a parking lot or some apartments to serve the needs of the city or county.

Political bureaucracy has, and will continue, to overwhelm health care services, and in turn will create a flood of premature deaths, a greater shortage of providers, and patients traveling to Mexico and other countries for these lost services. In comparing one bureaucracy (HMO/MCO) to another (government), the first is not cheaper than the latter. The difference might be that the 30%-40% which HMOs are now making come off of provider reimbursement rates. Making providers part of the civil service program might restrain those specialists, such as surgeons who make $5000 an hour, and the rest of the providers might welcome some sense of security and stability. In any change of management there are those who are happy and those who are unhappy. Currently those who are dissatisfied with the current changes are leaving the health care field, are working fewer hours, or are working under a public corporation, non-profit, or governmental organizations.

A single payer is a term used to mean that the government would run the health care system rather than paying HMOs and states to operate the administrative duties of such a program. If the federal government does take this next step, they will have nationalized the healthcare industry. There are those who argue that a universal health care system could be more effective and efficient than what the practice of medicine has been over the past century. Arnold S. Relman, MD argues that there is a need to change how we insure, how health care is financed, and the way it is organized and delivered. He suggests that a one-payer system could also allow those with private insurance to opt out of the national insurance coverage. Relman sees doctors working within multi-specialty, not-for-profit organizations and accepting a salary determined by the group management. The argument for national health coverage is spawned by the current cost of health care and how medical care has been "governed by commerce and private enterprise rather than by public regulation and social need" (Relman, 2007, p. 2).

Given recent communications from those that are part of the research for decision makers for the Department of Health and Human Services and/or the Centers for Medicare and Medicaid Services, they are already discussing openly that "eventually" this is where our country is headed.

The fight between state and federal government is likely to continue for the next twenty years, perhaps even forever. In the meantime, private practitioners of all disciplines will have to decide how to adjust to the antagonist programs. It is clear that we have many talented professionals who are putting in hours and hours of their time and energy, taking out student loans, only to find when they enter their practice, they are not able to receive the income they need that would warrant going in debt and investing years in educational advancement. The Internet is full of jobs that pay more and don't require as much education, thus alleviating student loans. The programs that trained welders, carpenters, and machinists, used to be called trade schools. Junior colleges can fund these programs cheaper than four-year universities. With the boom of oil fields in the United States, workers are recruited from non-degree personnel, and their starting pay is often 50% higher than psychologists, and twice as high as what first-year teachers receive.

Those who have invested their time, energy, and money in obtaining a master's or doctorate degree have to be asking themselves: what was I thinking? Many of those now in school are turning toward jobs that have fewer liabilities, no overhead expenses, a good pension, and benefits including more vacation time than they would receive in private or group practice. The next chapter discusses ways to return to the roots of health care; listening to people, learning from them, and problem solving.

Chapter Three

From Misfits to Managers

Changing hats in clinical practice from physician to business owner can be very uncomfortable; it is like being patient-centered in approach to clinical issues, and then having to manage irrational thoughts and behaviors in a business-like manner. This change in presentation to patients and their families has become a critical juncture for the state of private practice today and threatens its very existence. Within this chapter we will tackle the issue of management, which most providers have very little knowledge of unless they have been in private practice for over six years. While the number six is not a magic standard of time, it does imply; however, that learning the business side of practice takes time. The fact that one has an MBA and a PhD degree(s) does not necessarily imply competency in business management, organizing tax information, appointment scheduling, budgets, time management, policies, human resources, and risks and liabilities.

We can all recall starting college and feeling how great it was to be out of the nest, free to try new behaviors, to be reckless, uninhibited, and then being scared to death when actually trying these new behaviors. This feeling was like being out of place, out from the cover of protection of our families, and fighting the urge to reach out to our families and our security blanket of home. So it is with managing time, staff, and budgets. Even when we have taken graduate courses in management, it is easier to join a large organization and to be absorbed by the template of management routines and tasks. In private practice you create your own template and, unfortunately, that can be viewed as illegal or inadequate for justification of services.

Diversity of cultural and social values, new technology, unknown legislative acts, new enforcement agencies, a lack of communication between HMOs and providers, as well as between state Medicaid Administrators and providers, leaves most providers feeling isolated and detached. It is becoming harder for providers to start a private practice given the antagonistic attitude from HMO case managers and representatives with providers. Anyone considering forming a private practice should be committed to a long-term therapy relationship with a psychiatrist. Then there are the graduate professors who fail to offer the business side of practice and forget to warn of the dangers of being in a private practice. Therapists, as well as primary care physicians, psychiatrists, and psychologists, are trained to respond to the feelings of patients. With the growing managerial and business tasks that are forced on providers, they have to adjust to a transitional phase, such as a learning curve, which is often very awkward; perhaps the way a square peg feels when being shoved into a circular or rectangular hole.

TIME MANAGEMENT

Time is a resource and, as such, needs to be managed in the same way as do people, projects, and programs. It takes time to organize and effectively communicate the delegating of tasks to staff members or sharing tasks as partners. What is your time worth? If you make $60,000 per year, that translates into 52 cents a minute. When you add up the salaries of everyone in your practice, plus all the overhead costs not associated with payroll, it is possible that you might find that your business costs are over $100 per hour. If you can only bill an average of $50 per hour, then your business is in serious trouble, or you are in the wrong business. For mental health practitioners who have lost over 30% of reimbursement dollars and another 20% in restrictions of trade (restricting numbers of family services that can be billed per therapist), staying in private practice or group practice is impossible unless there are non-profit organizations or other institutions, such as government agencies, corporations, or hospitals, that can offer positions. Many are working six days a week, and often over 12 hours a day, and are continuing to lose money. If physicians were restricted the way mental health practitioners are currently being restricted, there would a severe shortage of primary care physicians.

There are several ways to manage time:

- Identification of daily tasks
- Realistic expectations of daily accomplishments
- Division of time between clinical and business (management) tasks
- Prioritize tasks
- Plan for the unexpected, such as no-shows
- Make sure to build in time for lunch

A clinician decides that a letter to a primary care physician is needed to update records on a patient and to suggest a medication or dosage evaluation, or possibly even a referral. Letter writing takes concentration and when patients are sitting there watching, they are apt to interfere or interject thoughts, which can be a distraction. Such distractions can lead to spelling errors as well as not communicating effectively. Therefore, alternatives include taking work home, staying late in the evenings, or working weekends. In any event, time is added to work and this time is then deducted from family time. Costs go up and revenues go down. The motivation for spending more time at work rather than at home is to improve your clinical practice. Neglecting families has its own costs.

The motivation for HMOs and MCOs to bid on the Medicaid population programs is the enormous pot of gold offered by states. They also see a window of opportunity, which will allow them to keep more of the Medicaid dollars, at least for the next six to ten years, because reimbursement rates of providers can be cut to the point that many will be driven out of large Medicaid regions, which, in turn, will lower the usage rate. As this happens the HMOs and MCOs can show how they have been able to cut Medicaid budgets. They are then rewarded for their efforts with a slice of the savings created through their reimbursement rate cuts and gatekeeper refusals. With President Obama's Affordable Care Act, one can expect that by the year 2014 millions of people will be entitled to health care benefits where once they were uninsured or underinsured. The Act is a way to increase accessibility to millions who have not had this coverage before. The conflict between the Act and the current efforts of state represent a political power play at the expense of patients who are seeing a gatekeeper position standing in the way of requested services, which were once available. This is a way for MCOs and HMOs to make additional income since patients living in rural communities will have to drive a great distance for services. It is unlikely they will do so because it will mean spending hours on a round trip to see a mental health care provider, or even a primary care physician. They are more likely to self-medicate, use emergency rooms (ERs), or resort to crime, or other self-destructive behavior, to release their anger, frustration, and pain, both emotional and physical. Only a sudden increase in rural health tragedies that will spotlight the results of the access problems has any hope of turning this picture around. The loss of lives alone will not be sufficient to build up a ground swell of support for change; it will have to be more dramatic and involve the national media. States and corporate executives are so entrenched into the U.S. Treasury pipeline that forcing a change will be difficult since they tend to have greater influence over judges, lawyers, and the systems of appeal than do patients or providers.

SCHEDULING

Software that allows scheduling every 30 minutes and that also has room for name, date of birth, phone number, and type of insurance can give the receptionist who pulls charts the necessary information in order to differentiate between patients with similar names. Keeping patient files in locked file cabinets is important for security, as well as confidentiality. The file cabinets should also be easily assessable to the one pulling files. The use of coloring schemes on patients' files can quickly differentiate between patients from different towns or to tell one type of case from another. At the end of the day all files should be placed in the locked cabinet, or on the biller's desk behind a locked door. At one practice patients used to sign in, now it is common to fine the receptionist if he/she has allowed others the opportunity to see the names of everyone that checked in that day. Along with scheduling, the receptionist should be prepared to print out the next appointment for the patient, as well as an excuse for school, work, or for proof of attendance for the Medicaid travel expense program.

POLICY ON NO-SHOWS

At one time patients would fail to come to their appointment without fear of consequences. Today, in many communities, physicians and allied professionals are charging a no-show fee that is collected at the next visit, or there may not be a next visit. The costs of these absences cost the practices thousands of dollars each year. If a practice has scheduled ten people for a Monday and only 5 show up, at a charge of $100, then the practice loses $500. If multiplied by 9 days out of the month, then the lost revenue for that one month was $4500. If all the patients are Medicaid patients and the fee per billable hour is $56, then the per day's loss would be $336. If the number of days were only nine for the month, then the loss would be $3024, a substantial amount for a small practice. If a practice is going to initiate such a fee, then patients must sign a statement so they can be aware of the policy, as well as the fees. Most practices instruct patients that in order to cancel an appointment, they must call in 24 hours PRIOR to the scheduled appointment. When people call the morning of the appointment, there will be a $25 fee for re-scheduling. This often has the effect of patients changing their plans to avoid the fee.

CONFIDENTIALITY

These are issues that often come up, especially when they fear others, who might read the file, would misinterpret the information or who might use it against them in some manner. Issues such as suicidal ideations, family violence, criminal activity, or substance abuse are the most frequent ones that people seem to want to protect. Therefore, confidentiality needs to be addressed during the initial assessment. A form with the patient's signature, which is completed prior to the initial assessment, is important in documenting the discussion of this issue.

Now more than ever, health care providers need to set aside at least $10,000 for legal representation, with the understanding that it will take approximately another $20,000 for representation against any allegation of insurance fraud. If a patient accuses a provider of a lack of competence, an unethical relationship, misrepresenting their credentials, or breaking confidence, then legal representation is normally supplied by the professional liability insurance company. Normally, the licensing board hears these cases. When a complaint is filed, a certified letter is sent to the provider who then has 15 days to submit a reply. When the letter is received, the prudent provider will notify his/her professional liability insurance company. They will need to see all the papers sent by the licensing board including the complaint and the provider's response. Within a short period of time the company will call with the name and phone number of the attorney appointed for the provider's representation.

> Confidentiality is critical to the therapist-client relationship, for that reason, it also is the areas in which the therapist is exposed to the greatest liability. The range of confidentiality extends from the content of a therapy session to the fact that a given client is being seen. Although it is no less sacred to them than the priest's Seal of Confession, therapists now are asked more frequently to violate their mandate of client confidentiality. The reasons are myriad, including court action, potentially dangerous clients, and professional impropriety (Earle, Barnes, 1999, pp. 111-112).

One reason confidentiality creates problems for therapists and patients is that governmental programs like HIPAA were created to encourage confidentiality, but at the same time the payer of insurance claims has the ability to sell health information to life insurance companies, and any other insurance company that requests the information. This is one of the most fundamental weaknesses with relationships to MCOs and HMOs.

> Details about highly personal matters are routinely sent off to managed care companies and insurance companies. At the same time, managed care companies are going through great upheavals in ownership. So what? Suppose you are sending confidential material to the XYZ Managed Care Company, which has convinced you that it knows how to safeguard such information properly. What happens to that material when the company is purchased by ABC Managed Care, whose standards or practices might be radically different? When

we release highly private information about people, we lose control over it (Ackley, 1997, p. 53).

In 2005, Kaiser Permanente paid a $200,000 fine for leaving sensitive patient information on a public accessible website. According to published reports, data, which included lab results of 150 patients, was posted for more than a year. Between February 2005 and October 2006, nearly 350 breaches occurred at corporations, institutions, and government agencies in the United States, resulting in 93.7 million records containing sensitive personal data being compromised, according to the Privacy Rights Clearinghouse, a not-for-profit organization in San Diego, California.

> One of the most important rights included in HIPAA is the right to obtain copies of your medical records. HIPAA also allows you to ask to change inaccurate information in your medical records. For more on your right to access medical records under HIPAA, see PRC Fact Sheet 8a, HIPAA Basics: Medical Privacy in the Electronic Age, www.privacyrights.org/fs/fs8a-hipaa.htm. See the sample letter for requesting a copy of your medical records, www.privacyrights.org/Letters/medical2.htm (Privacy Rights Clearinghouse, 2008).

When exploring the Privacy Rights Clearinghouse website, most people might be shocked by how many companies are formed to monitor not only credit reports but specialty reports. These can include medical history (Medical Information Bureau report); history of your housing payments (Rent Bureau); check writing history, including bounced checks (ChexSystems); employment background, which is often checked during an application for employment (LexisNexis Screening Solutions); and homeowner and auto insurance claims (CLUE reports). The Fair Credit Reporting Act (FCRA) covers financial health history, but it can include more, such as reports made to employers, insurance companies, banks, and landlords. To learn more about your credit reporting rights, see PRC Fact Sheet 6, *How Private Is My Credit Report?* at www.privacyrights.org/fs/fs6-crdt.htm.

As the federal government pushes for more collaboration between health care providers, the loss of control of health care information is likely to grow. Consider the case of the rogue employee who exposes health care information after being fired. Or the problems generated by outsourced billing services, or even letters faxed between providers on patients. Faxes are not always safe, even when a statement is placed on the form in regards to compliance with the Health Insurance Portability Accountability Act of 1996. This law has a weakness when outlining legal action that can be taken by an individual or a corporation with an angry ex-employee. Companies are taking steps to protect their businesses by creating a privacy officer who will set standards of information security, investigate any allegations of leaks or a break in standards, increase training of employees, and determine discipline for employees. This whole field of medical identity theft is growing up all around us, and so are the security companies that specialize in identity theft, credit care theft, corporate secrets, and insurance information theft. As more medical data goes online, the risk of a breach goes up.

Poor administrative decision making can also lead to a breakdown in compliance. Such was the case of the Prime Health Care Services Hospital in Redding, California. The hospital CEO was reported to have sent an e-mail to 785 employees of the hospital that disclosed a patient's confidential medical files. The CEO felt compelled to disclose information that proved, in the hospital administration's eyes, that they had provided adequate information and treatment in regards to a particular patient's illness. A California Watch news report accused them of contributing to an outbreak of a Third World nutritional disorder in the hospital (Williams, 2012). Health care privacy concerns are going global. For an update of the efforts to protect health care information in the United States as well as the world, Google Deborah C. Peel, MD and read what she has written about health care privacy issues.

ECONOMICS OF THERAPY

The business side of health care includes the use of mission and vision statements, management tasks, strategies in marketing, advertising, administrative tasks, such as billing and collections, human resource management responsibilities, managing the financial books (accounts payable, accounts receivable), analyzing tax strategies and financial statements, and Profit & Loss Statements (P&Ls), with balance sheets. Without experience in balancing budgets and forecasting, the mission and vision statements are meaningless bits of information. Businesses operate on capital and revenue streams. When you only have one revenue stream, you place the company in a very vulnerable economic position. With what we know about business cycles and patterns of tension between demand and supply, managers can be expected to stay up at night working out "what if" scenarios (such as, in the event you lose a panel position you will need to replace those time slots with another revenue stream or cut expenses. For example, working five days each week instead of six). What if your company was audited and the material requested could take you weeks to sit down and analyze the allegations. What do you do? Would your practice shut down during this time? If so, are the fees the recoupment or insurer auditors demand worth the time and effort to take so much time off in order to fight the allegations? Balance that against the cost of an attorney for representation with the board. When one source collapses, a good manager has another source waiting in the wings.

The business of therapy, or health care, is also about the economy of that business within the marketplace. One of the reporting companies that collects information about the financial history of companies and corporations is called Dun and Bradstreet, which has been stocking commercial information for over 170 years. Currently their database has information on 200 million businesses globally. They offer risk management features that include predictive indicators of financial health, which can streamline credit requests. Dun and Bradstreet accumulate credit and risk information from a variety of sources; their databases offer information about:

- Public company records from: U.S. courts & state offices; business registrations, suits, liens & judgment filings; UCC filings; bankruptcy filings
- Private company info/financials: detailed on the largest U.S. firms, financial statements & basics on millions more
- Credit & supplier risk scores based on more than 110M accounts receivable records accessed through our unique Trade Reporting Program (Dun and Bradstreet, 2012)

If a private practice operates as a company, with incorporation or with the use of a personal name or a DBA (doing business as), when applying for a business loan, or when applying for a contract with a state or federal agency (i.e., state corrections system), there is often a requirement for a Dun and Bradstreet member number. This number is obtained by going to Dun and Bradstreet and completing information about your company or corporation. They will provide a number that represents your company on Dun and Bradstreet, and the report will provide information to the government about your financial health, which may have either a negative or a positive impact on a bank loan or contract bid/application.

   Economics is part of the economy of business. Some terms that are often common language for small businesses include:

- Supply and demand—this means that a business of any size can be affected by the demands of customers and the amount of goods kept in stock, or the services that a health care provider can offer.
- Economics—the study of the production of goods or services available to meet the demands of the public and the resources available to create the goods and services demanded.
- Economies of scale—the tug-of-war with diseconomies of scale that defines the average costs of a product or service over a long-run that leads to an increase or decrease of all imputes in the manufacturing of products, or the creation of services offered for sale. When studied, this information can suggest the length of life of the product or service in a community.

- Absolute poverty—the term used to define the amount of income a person or family needs in order to purchase the absolute minimum basic necessities of life. These basic necessities are identified in terms of calories of food, BTUs of energy, square feet of living space, and medical costs. The problem with this term is that there are no absolutes and when it comes to survival, not one family is an average family. Economists and researchers often use these terms, when it is relative to providers of health care to determine if they wish to work in communities where there is a higher level of economic poverty. Sometimes economic poverty suggests educational poverty, but this is not always the case. The lack of education usually refers to formal education; not informal or street survival skills. Educated people can lose their jobs and still meet economic poverty levels.
- Elasticity—This term responds to changes in one variable (usually quantity demanded or quantity supplied) compared to changes in another variable (usually demand price or supply price). When the anticipated changes in health care reform are fully implemented, forecasters have reported that millions of people will then be covered by some type of both medical and mental health insurance. This anticipation is causing changes within managed care and state budgets and has an effect on the areas of the country that have shortages of health care providers. The demands for health services are expected to grow given this scenario. How it will affect the typical provider largely depends on where their practice is within the state and if they are willing to accept the Medicaid HMOs. While it may seem like the Golden Goose has landed, state officials are already cutting reimbursement rates and are having their Solicitor General "red flag" providers that are providing above the average for a license or billing code, and then institute audits to challenge their financial strengths as well as their internal fortitude to continue to practice in a fee-for-service arena. This means when the audit comes down, and you respond to it with documentation, within a short period of time the Solicitor General's office will send a recoupment bill stating that they estimate the provider has been overpaid on the billing dates that were sent to him/her and that they have thirty days to send a complete check. Most providers may not be able to accommodate this demand and if they cannot pay up in thirty days, each billing that they send to Medicaid or an HMO will take the reimbursement check and apply it on the provider's account. When the payment is paid in full, plus interest, then the provider can start receiving checks. In the meantime the provider must have the financial means to keep the office open and the operating and payroll checks current. If not, they tend to close their practices. There is no appeal process until all the fees have been paid and the appeal process is geared to be rejected at the state level and at the federal level according to state legislators' aides.

- Opportunity costs—The comparison of cost in regards to the opportunity to purchase, to accept a loan, or to expand a business vs. the cost of not accepting the opportunity at that point in time.
- Competitive edge—This term suggests that one or more parties have an edge in professional status (license), education, financial and/or political positioning in the community, or years of experience.
- Interest—The amount a bank charges for providing a loan service. When considering a location for a practice, the cost per square foot should be compared in different parts of the city or county. Those near financial institutions or hospitals will be more expensive than those in a smaller shopping center. The cost of one location vs. another is often more than the accessibility to a population a practice wishes to attract, but also includes the type of financing available from banking institutions. An example of this is when comparison is made of the costs of purchasing a car vs. the interest received if the money were kept in a savings account. Comparison should be made of the interest rate of the loan to the interest rate of savings, which may influence a business decision.
- Marketplace—The place where business is performed in exchange for currency or credit. Markets are also a place where business people and entities discuss business ventures and projects.
- Capital—The currency or exchange between a buyer and seller that has economic value to both.
- Human capital—Typically the value of employees to the service or product that is being marketed.
- Financial capital—The financial resources available to an individual or business.
- Physical capital—Buildings, warehouses, office space, equipment, and furnishings owned by a company.
- Social capital—The reputation of an individual or company in a community.
- Gross Domestic Deficit (GDD)—The estimated sum of all economic activities in a country over a period of twelve months.
- Credit and Debit—Banking terms: when money is deposited into a bank account it's a credit; when a check is written on the account it's a debit.

A business, of any size, is created to make money for the owner or stockholders. For health care providers this has been a point of internal conflict as many providers will enter the field of service for the passion they have for the process; making money is not a top priority. The risks and liabilities of being a licensed entity in the health care industry today are putting enormous pressure on providers to rethink their level of commitment. They are now finding out how easy it is for governmental agencies, working in collaboration with MCOs and HMOs, to force providers to accept conditions of participation on panels including controlling more and more of their daily functions while reducing revenues. This places providers in a vulnerable position where they cannot even afford to defend themselves against the giants of industry. Patients will begin to pay the price for the relationship between the MCOs, HMOs, and government. Many will find their providers will not accept either the state or federal programs, and they might be closing their doors to all patients. This is the power of economic and political leverage.

Cycles of business refers to the effects of supply and demand. As jobs are lost, people back off from purchases, such as vacations, cars, travel, and entertainment. If it is necessary to travel to see a specialist, and Medicaid refuses to pay travel costs, patients will not go for treatments or medications. This is why many people have used ERs for office visits, due to the fact that they have no insurance and no money. Private practices that see children for school testing and other events, often keep the children from making a doctor's appointment. School testing days are known events that prohibit, in most cases, children being released from school to see a doctor or therapist. At the start of every school year, obtain a copy of all testing days and holidays within that year.

Then there are cycles of natural disasters. Although they do not hit every year, they can be expected during any given year to take patients away from the office. They could also cause more patients to come into the office with complaints of insomnia, nightmares, and flashbacks.

Business cycles fluctuate similarly to how shoppers spend more during some times of the year than at other times, such as the Christmas holidays compared to the first two weeks in February. In other words, you can depend on fluctuations, cycles, and no-shows at the most inopportune time for your practice. Guarding against these times of lower or higher income may require a lot of thinking in the quiet hours of the morning, and planning during the day for those rocky financial times. Getting a flood of patients can be even more stressful than not getting enough and this can also disrupt the flow of income because now you may have to work an extra day, or put in evening hours, or hire a part-time staff member to help with the paperwork.

HUMAN RESOURCES

Mental health care providers are finding positions in non-profit organizations, schools, governmental agencies, mixed medical group services, or in private practices. Many providers may never have to worry about hiring and firing employees. Of those who do, understanding the different laws that affect a practice or corporation is critical. Human resources refers to employees of a company. Human resource managers are those responsible for managing employee support services. The Human Resource Department provides the framework for developing employee skills, knowledge and interpersonal skills, and communications. Human resource personnel are responsible for performance development and management, coaching employees, training employees, key employee identification process, and organizational development programs. They assist managers and directors in discipline as well as reward programs. This department is responsible for writing job descriptions which tell employees what they were hired for, how much they will be paid, what hours they will work, details about lunch time, insurance and sick day benefits, and how their position fits into the rest of the organization. Those responsible for human resource tasks need to study how others before them wrote the job tasks, how the tasks and positions were analyzed, and definitions of specific terms for those positions. Such tasks add up to the value of that position, steps of pay increases, licenses and college degrees needed, and if there are other duties or levels of experience needed to qualify for a position. With this information the staff can write an advertisement for the print media, or write a description of needs of the organization for a "headhunter" who searches banks of resumes and vitas for a match and then does the preliminary interview with the prospective employee.

The HR department, or individual private practitioner, also has the responsibility to ensure the organization is aware of, and in compliance with, state and federal regulations. We work and live within a very litigious society. Every human resource director or manager needs to be conferring with an attorney that understands and works with human resource issues. This is important because there are a number of different legal issues that a corporation or a small business owner needs to know in order to make decisions within the law that affect employees. Here are a few:

- American Disability Act
- Equal Opportunity
- Family and Medical Leave Act
- Employees who are in the armed forces.
- Hostile environment issues
- Employee terminations
- Occupational Safety and Health Act (OSHA)
- HIPAA
- Consolidated Omnibus Budget Reconciliation Act of 1986 (COBRA)—for gaps in insurance coverage
- Discrimination issues
- Worker's Compensation

Some programs that the human resource manager may take a lead in:

- Job task analyses
- Writing job descriptions
- Writing want ads
- Recruitment
- Testing
- Creating forms and a filing system
- Updating the employee manual
- Administration of employee benefits and compensation packages

One can easily understand how a person in private practice who wishes to hire staff or contract labor, or who hopes to begin a group practice, needs to be familiar with these regulations, state and federal programs, and the tasks expected of a human resource manager. Most small business owners take on more than they realize at first, as they only think of expansion from a singular position; however, taking on employees is a major commitment of time and resources that are seldom contemplated prior to making some decisions regarding expansion. Many times small business owners see that they are too busy to do certain things and so they look for someone to help them. Many times skills needed for positions in an office are not readily available in rural and border communities, which is why many health care providers never give moving to these locations a second thought.

A painful example of this last point was the hiring of an office manager in a two-man operation, where one was the owner and the other one was the part time contract person. When the office manager was first hired, information about her past was never validated and therefore the owner never knew about the felony for welfare fraud. For the first two years things went along pretty well until one day she got jealous of a new part-time clerk/filer and offered to help the office's contract therapist by turning over files that belonged to the owner; the contractor offered to pay her $50 per file. This went on for a number of months when another unethical trait surfaced. She overheard the business owner say something about the difficult nature of a young man he was seeing. Instead of keeping this information confidential, she called the mother of the boy and revealed what she had heard. The mother stormed into the office threatening to sue. When the owner found out, he fired the office manager, after which the second employee told him of the special relationship between the office manager and the contract therapist. The former office manager filed for worker's compensation, which was granted by the Texas Work Force Commission because "there was no violation of any law including HIPAA." For several years she rode the unemployment ticket, which cost the owner thousands of dollars.

When the owner audited the files of the former contract therapist a few months later, he found that the office manager had been accepting incomplete progress forms from the contract therapist and billing for them. There were 52 incomplete progress forms signed by the contract therapist. A complaint was filed with the licensing board, and a letter with progress note names was turned over to the Medicaid Integrity Department. The owner had to repay for the 52 cases, thus losing more money. The Medicaid department never went after the contract therapist. The therapist was able to drag the complaint out for two years before he was suspended. He was then reinstated within 30 days. Today he still practices in Texas.

The cost of doing business can become huge and the experiences ugly. The negative energy of contesting unemployment benefits or going to licensing boards to fight complaints from disgruntled former employees drains positive energy from practice owners. It is difficult for those in private practice and small group practices to afford a quality human resource program, but without it they should not be hiring staff. They could outsource human resource tasks, which may be a cheaper alternative. Hiring legal staff to do these chores would not be cost effective. Hiring an attorney to create employment contracts would be more helpful for the honest person than for those who are looking to sabotage a competitor. The fact that one has a professional license is no guarantee of ethical work habits, as the case above demonstrates.

Unemployment insurance is paid out of a corporation's 941 Schedule Form each quarter. This insurance helps pay unemployment benefits to employees who are laid off. In accordance with the Workforce Commission in each state, there are reasons for refusing unemployment benefits to employees that have been terminated. Under federal guidelines, states provide benefits based on the length of time on the job. The purpose of unemployment insurance is to provide workers, who are unemployed through no fault of their own, with monetary payments for a specific time period or until the worker finds a new job. In many cases, the compensation will be half of the individual's earnings, up to a maximum amount. For example:

> In New York State you're entitled to collect up to a maximum of $405, which is half the state's average weekly wage while in Arizona, the highest benefit rate is $205. The maximum benefit in California is $450 and the average weekly unemployment benefit for all states is $293. The Internal Revenue Service counts unemployment insurance benefits as income, so your check is taxable. Depending on the state, state and federal income tax can be withheld from your check (Alison Doyle, 2012).

Termination of an employee needs to show documentation of counseling prior to termination. The Workforce Commission may vary from state to state, but insubordination is one of the major reasons for termination. Making unsubstantiated statements can lead to an investigation from the state Workforce Commission with assistance from the state's Attorney General. Having witnessed this firsthand, the CEO who used an employee to manufacture reasons for termination, faces the possibility of jail time, as well as loss of his CEO position in his non-profit organization. Consulting legal representation that specializes in this type of case is worth the time and the fees in order to ensure your company is in line with state law.

RISK MANAGEMENT

The health care reform movement has been growing for decades, working through various elements of resistance, showing its face around corners, other times appearing off stage just out of camera range. In the past few years it has been more forward, boldly stepping into the light, even staring into the camera's eye as if waiting to see who will blink first. With the reform movement, an entourage of lobbyists, special interest groups, and members of the Wall Street family has appeared. Since the Twin Towers terrorist attacks was an assault on Americans on the soil of the United States, politicians have fought over camera time to pledge alliance to the flag and to their faith. Then they walk off camera to huddle with committees and special interest groups to fight over the American dollar. Since the Bush Wars and the development of the United States Department of Homeland Security, DHS as a cabinet department of the United States federal government, there has been a rush of spin-off contracts with Halliburton, Kellogg, Brown & Root, Vinnell, Brown & Root, General Electric, Bechtel Group, Fluor Group, Louis Berger Group, Boeing, Blackwater USA, Lockheed Martin, Northrop Grumman, General Dynamics, Raytheon, United Technologies, Science Applications International Corporation, and CSC/DynCorp. These are just a few of the general contractors that were awarded contracts that were worth billions of dollars in Kuwait, Iraq, Afghanistan, and Turkey (Chatterjee, 2003). Some are still working contracts in that region, as well as in central Asian countries. DHS has more than 200,000 employees with their stated mission to protect the air, water, and land space of the United States. Another agency with significant homeland security responsibilities is the Departments of Health and Human Services, Justice, and Energy. In 2011 the federal government allotted this department $98 million and they spent $67 million. Risk management for a security system means creating awareness of the many ways the United States can be attacked. In financial institutions risk management means assessing and quantifying business risks, then taking measures to control or reduce them. In health care, practicing risk management means assessing exposures to financial losses, legal actions, and ethical standard violations, and then assessing and quantifying them and taking steps to avoid or reduce the exposure.

By numbers alone, large corporations, such as hospitals, have the greatest risk for liabilities; however, they also have the greatest number of revenue streams that allow them to retain legal teams, consultants, and lobbyists to insulate them. In comparison, private practitioners of any discipline have the greatest exposure since they have the lowest amount of funds available to protect and insulate their practice and their investments. While primary care physicians who train and hire physician assistants and family nurse practitioners can generate greater revenues, they can lose it all with a high profile court case, or a charge of money laundering and/or insurance fraud, or bringing medications to the United States from Mexico and then charging Medicaid and Medicare. While this last allegation has hurt some primary care physicians along the border, some have remained in practice because their practices were so large it allowed them to sustain sizeable legal fees and penalties.

Legislative laws often bring changes that miss the eyes of private practitioners but would never fly past large corporations, such as hospitals, because their wealth allows them to hire people to specifically watch each bill in state and federal legislatures and then analyze them for application and relevance in regards to their corporation. For example, a piece of legislation passed in the Texas legislature in 2009 did not affect practices until 2011, when the Solicitor General turned the gun on mental health private practices. The result is likely to be 500 or more private practitioners closing their practices and moving into non-profits, educational institutions, or into the field of coaching. Most, if not all, of these practices are in areas already short of mental health providers and services. The legislation included parts that applied to billing for family therapy. The legislation turned bill stated that only one billable hour a day could be billed for family therapy per family. While on the surface this may sound rational, when applied to each case, it hurts cliental practice. Now after 45 to 50 minutes, families have to stop therapy, even though they might be at a breakthrough moment, go home, and return another time without having closure of issues and completion of assessments. Those that wrote the bill were administrative personnel, some with licenses such as RN or MD and they are on the staff of the state Medicaid organization or the Solicitor General's office. Their allegiance is as clear as is their bias, which distorts their professional vision and judgment. State legislators, when questioned, did not know about this portion of the bill. As in most cases, legislative assistants are hired to read bills and then to translate them for the legislators. Someone missed the boat this time. Now over 500 therapists are having their reimbursement checks kidnapped and used to pay back thousands of dollars. When asked about an appeal process, the Solicitor General's office said that any appeal has to be AFTER the money is returned to the state. Then there is an opaque system of appeal that weighs heavily on the size of the government and makes it virtually impossible to recoup the funds. If the American judicial system operated this way, those accused of crimes, such as murder, would have to serve their time or be executed first before they could appeal. But isn't the Solicitor General's office part of the Texas Attorney General's office? Isn't that part of the judicial system? Big Brother has become so powerful that they can usurp traditional processes such as judicial fairness and organizational communication, which teaches that important changes within the organization are communicated first with all of the departments and then with all of the employees; however, the 2009 legislation was printed in some Medicaid bulletins on the Internet. Something large corporations would have had read by a committee, but for private practice owners there would have been no time or assistance in finding, reading, then having translated the bill into non-legal language. With the letters sent out to these chosen providers, there was a bit of information that sounded like a school report card: you have exceeded billing of family therapy hours beyond the average of those with the same license. The second percentage number stated that I out billed more than the average person with the same license. Wow! Thanks, I'm successful. People besides my patients are acknowledging my efforts!

But I hardly think they meant it as a complement; why else would they ask me to return thousands of dollars to the Texas coffer? In reality, this is all part of the Texas Governor's efforts to lower the state budget. He is the reverse of Robin Hood. He takes from the have-nots and gives to the haves and calls it helping the poor do their part to lower the state budget. They can, and do, get away with this because who can fight Goliath? If little David with his sling shot were alive, he would not have been allowed to carry a bag of rocks onto the battlefield because the rocks and sling-shot were not issued items for battle.

> Traditionally, risk management was thought of as mostly a matter of getting the right insurance. Insurance coverage usually comes in rather standard packages, so people tended to not take risk management seriously. However, this impression of risk management has changed dramatically. With the recent increase in rules and regulations, employee-related lawsuits and reliance on key resources, risk management is becoming a management practice that is every bit as important as financial or facilities management (Free Management Library, 2012).

In health care, like homeland security, risk management is a key player in the growth of the company as well as the security. Those with a romantic twinkle in their eye should re-think private practice and look for a larger umbrella to operate within in order to have time to learn all the nuances of health care laws, regulations, and enforcement agencies. No one enters health care without spending or investing a lot of time, energy, and money in their educational preparation for this profession.

Among the many things we can learn from the business side of health care services is that medical and allied health care providers are playing catch-up to those who make a living to make as much money as they can, which often means using a network of political and corporate contacts to obtain favored status when both state and federal governments are passing out contracts. Providers and scholars presented a number of subjects in an effort to encourage further studies. The business terms presented were not intended to be all-inclusive. Time management is important for scheduling as well as a technique to keep on task. Providers often are multi-tasking people and can, at times, forget details, miss deadlines, and step away from a project before completion. The biggest irritants in regards to scheduling are the no-shows; those who forget their appointments. This adds costs to the practice regardless of whether it is a private practice, group practice, or a large corporation. Time is money, as the saying goes, and this is certainly the case for private practices since they are normally operating on a narrow margin of profit.

This chapter has provided a number of examples of risks and liabilities to a practice. Hospitals and large corporations often have a Director of Risk Management. One of the risks to a company is the loss of a revenue stream. If a panel spot is lost, they can no longer see people with that particular insurance, which means a loss of income since patients with that coverage are waiting to see you. Another risk that providers often push aside is the need for legal advice and guidance. Providers do this because they do not have the margins to pay legal fees. These individuals need to leave private practice and join a larger organization or institution that can provide the legal coverage needed. The next chapter covers threats to autonomy and the various hats that a provider-entrepreneur wears within a private practice.

Chapter Four

Redefining the Niche

This chapter discusses the identity of the provider within the practice of the community it serves. Finding your place in the community is an important part of defining your business. In most cases one's personal identity is developed by one's internal sense of who one is as a human, as a man or woman, and as a professional. The growth of personal awareness, of one's strengths and limitations, presents opportunities to maximize our assets and control or change our bad habits. This whole book is about how the past has been replaced by the future and how providers are the primary targets for solving the health care cost crisis. The fewer providers there are, the fewer bills that will be sent to HMOs, and the lower the cost of health care budgets for states. At one time providers offered techniques and services to either heal or to teach patients how to regain self-regulation and thus be able to change their lives into productive ones. Today providers are being used to solve state budgets.

In the 21st century not only do we face political and economic influences on our lives with our communities, but this is also coming from global markets. Events from Egypt, China, and New Zealand can be in our living rooms when we turn on the morning news. Foreign stock markets can influence the patterns of profit taking or the direction of investments on the New York Stock Exchange long before New Yorkers have had their first cup of java. To put the health care reform movement into perspective, there was no such movement prior to 50 years ago. That means that this new invention of ideas has been in our lifetime, as has the invention of television, talking movies, and the space program; we've seen an explosion of new medications, medical testing, and scanning devices that can address symptoms earlier than previous detection devices in America's history.

During the past 30 years the mental health field has expanded and contributed to the cost of health care. Also contributing to the cost of health care are medical inventions and new techniques such as transplants, new heart valves, re-attachment of limbs, reconstructive surgery, and the healing of certain diseases, which used to mean certain death, such as cancer, AIDS, pneumonia, polio, tuberculosis, malaria, and infections. In regards to mental health, the human behavioral theories of the 1960s opened up the field of talk therapy. They took away the couch and replaced it with chairs where face-to-face dialogue offered quicker opportunities in reaching solutions to problems as compared to the laborious psychoanalytic style of psychotherapy that few people could afford. In the 1950s there was a great shortage of psychologists, but today graduate schools have produced more master level therapists than doctorate level therapists. Therapists operate on the front lines of mental health along with the primary care physicians so the collaboration movement is nothing new to those who have been operating this way for the past 30 years. This brief perspective puts into focus the effects of the rapid growth on knowledge and experience in the health care profession, and the mental health segment of this industry is a vital player.

Private practices of health care, both medical and mental, are victims of an aggressive fight for the revenues they generate. The current winners are HMOs who are in an eating frenzy with millions of new Medicaid patients gained through a state lottery system for the prized business. Now the new managed care process begins to build in case managers as filters to services; new gatekeepers with a smile but with similar goals: cut costs to increase revenues for the HMOs and for their partner state(s). This is the business and the political sides of health care in which few physicians, chiropractors, nurses, psychologists, psychotherapists, physical therapists, and other providers have adequate knowledge. Lobbyists for the AMA and Wall Street corporations, including the Pharmaceutical Industry, now run both the political and business sectors of health care. The political awareness factor in mental health lags behind the physicians who are finding members to run for political offices. Physicians have held positions in Congress for years and more are running for office now due to the fact that they have watched as attorneys and business leaders have made laws affecting their lives and practices and they are tired of others determining their needs and what is good for the practice of health care. Mental health providers, as well as nurses, have been more reluctant to take those first political steps.

ALARM SOUNDED OVER THE SHORTAGES OF MENTAL HEALTH PROVIDERS

The following is a summary of a research study prepared for the Substance Abuse and Mental Health Services Administration (SAMHSA) by The Annapolis Coalition on the Behavioral Health Workforce (Cincinnati, Ohio) under Contract Number 280-02-0302 with SAMHSA, U.S. Department of Health and Human Services (DHHS).

> Most critically, there are significant concerns about the capability of the workforce to provide quality care. The majority of the workforce is uninformed about and unengaged in health promotion and prevention activities. Too many in the workforce also lack familiarity with resilience-and recovery-oriented practices and are generally reluctant to engage children, youth, and adults, and their families, in collaborative relationships that involve shared decision making about treatment options. It takes well over a decade for proven interventions to make their way into practice, since prevention and treatment services are driven more by tradition than by science. The workforce lacks the racial diversity of the populations it serves and is far too often insensitive to the needs of individuals, as these are affected by ethnicity, culture, and language. In large sections of rural America, there simply is no mental health or addictions workforce.

> There is overwhelming evidence that the behavioral health workforce is not equipped in skills or in numbers to respond adequately to the changing needs of the American population. While the incidence of co-occurring mental and addictive disorders among individuals has increased dramatically, most of the workforce lacks the array of skills needed to assess and treat persons with these co-occurring conditions. Training and education programs largely have ignored the need to alter their curriculum to address this problem and, thus, the nation continues to prepare new members of the workforce who simply are underprepared from the moment they complete their training.

It is difficult to overstate the magnitude of the workforce crisis in behavioral health. The vast majority of resources dedicated to helping individuals with mental health and substance abuse problems are human resources, estimated at over 80% of all expenditures (Blankertz & Robinson, 1997a). As this report documents, there is substantial and alarming evidence that the current workforce lacks adequate support to function effectively and is also largely unable to deliver care of proven effectiveness in partnership with the people who already need the services. There is equally compelling evidence of an anemic pipeline of new recruits to meet the complex behavioral health needs of the growing and increasingly diverse population in this country. The improvement of care, as well as the transformation of systems of care, depends entirely on a workforce that is adequate in size and effectively trained and supported (Hoge, Michael A., Morris, John A., Daniels, Allen S., Stuart, Gail W., Huey, Leighton Y., and Adams, Neal, 2007).

It should be noted that this was before the ACT was introduced and before the states reacted to implementation plans within HMOs to administer and monitor the providers of the Medicaid and Medicare population. If this study were to be updated, mental health providers would be less likely to be seen, not only in rural communities, but in all communities. This report documents many of the problems with the behavioral health workforce but says nothing about the problems in regards to access with this workforce or about all the cuts and recoupment actions against this workforce. When put together, the reader gets a clearer picture of the devastation of the behavioral health workforce over time, and also in terms of recent actions to prepare for the millions entering the Medicaid system in 2014. With the recent focus on improving the quality and quantity of the behavioral health workforce, due primarily from the volume of mass killings during 2012, future researchers and think tank specialists would do well to consider the issues presented within this book.

CHANGES IN THE PRACTICE DEVELOPMENT

The role of health care providers is changing as the demand for accountability and cost effectiveness is argued in the halls of legislatures. The roles played by those in private practice have changed due to sources in corporate office as well as by the suggestions from lobbyists representing special interest groups in corporate America. Case managers and area representatives are presenting to private practitioners ways in which they need to change. If they do not then the HMOs can call in the Solicitor General to audit their files and "find" evidence of some irregularity along with perhaps "failure to justify" a session or two. They might then make an "estimate" which would cause the "billing error" to be rectified with a payback of $10,000 before the provider can continue receiving reimbursements and before the appeal process can kick in.

HMOs have a direct influence on hours of operation, number of billings per day, reimbursement rates, new regulations, and new mandatory working relationships. As our professional roles are being reshaped, this has an impact on our relationships with families and friends. Those considering investing in a private practice for the future need to be aware of how the development of a practice is going to be affected by the new Accountability Act. Putting up a shingle with an impressive title and degree on an office door may have meant something 50 years ago, but in today's marketplace there has to be a new development process. Developing one's place in the profession and in the community refers to how a health care provider wants to be known, how one chooses to set up a practice, and what services your practice offers. When people say your name, an image is created instantly within their brain. That image is part of how a provider wants to be known.

Another problem facing providers is the number of people that do not keep their appointments. A recent Gallup Poll reveals that 55% of those who do not have insurance postpone doctor appointments. "This problem of delayed treatment, which is bad for patient health and physician revenue alike, is not limited to the uninsured. Thirty percent of the privately insured are care postponers compared with 21% of Americans receiving Medicare or Medicaid" (Lowes, Robert, 2012).

Their niche defines the specific services that a provider offers within defined demographics. Providers are defined by their services. Defining their market identity by a term such as psychologist, psychotherapist, counselor, or social worker will narrow down the population they serve. This tends to mainstream health care demands, which can be high or low depending on the awareness of the population served and the value of the services to their needs (personal and family). Narrow demographics tend to lead to elevated prices except for health care services, which are determined by a state's Medicaid administration, the federal Medicare administration, and the MCOs and HMOs. Therefore, if you are one of the few within a wide region, you can charge what you like, but contracts with the insurance administration (MCOs, HMOs, Medicaid and Medicare) will determine what you receive. As long as insurance contracts are accepted, the provider is obligated to abide by them or lose their contract to treat the patients carrying the insurance card. For example, products found in flea markets fluctuate in price as the demands for products and their availability increase or decrease. Not so for health care businesses. While there is a market for accepting just cash, these businesses tend to flourish in metropolitan regions, in which more upper level payrolls are found and where educational levels tend to be higher than in rural and border communities. Choosing to practice in a rural community due to the need is a good reason; however, there are many negatives that should be considered as well, such as isolation from colleagues, mentors, and those who may be needed for consultations as well as referral sources and/or sounding boards. Providers in mental health professions have a higher suicide rate than other professions. A majority of patients will have Medicaid, which is the lowest reimbursement rate. Finally, when working in a rural community, there is a tendency to be a generalist and not a specialist, which will widen the niche audience but will also open up the flood gates to difficult cases, a lack of community resources, and inadequate time and energy to do everything.

Positioning in a marketplace can mean the difference between just breaking even and making billions of dollars. Look how grocery stores position candy and tabloids near the checkout counter in order to promote impulse buying. Improving the sense of value in the health care marketplace can mean substantial revenues to mental health providers and can help in discussions of reimbursement rates. Some clinical psychologists have expanded their practices with the license to write prescriptions for a number of medications. At the same time, other psychologists have started a movement to promote how much more educated they are than those who do not have a doctorate degree, but instead have a certification from an American Psychology Association (APA) approved program and have coined a term to emphasize their superiority: sub doctorate level. Also, nurses have gained access to psychology courses and are now chosen over non-nursing licenses to direct many behavioral health programs in hospitals and also in some outpatient clinics. These issues between degree programs and licenses have become one of the contributors to the rift within the mental health community. It has created a stumbling block in efforts to unify what might lead to solidification and in turn to a stronger force and voice in legislative halls. The managed care organizations understand the value of leverage, and as long as the different degrees and licenses in mental health are disorganized and are building up boundaries to keep each other from the feeding trough, mental health providers will never realize their full potential at the negotiation table or with any political entity. The point has been made of how the business of therapy is not the only Achilles heel in the mental health segment of the health care industry; the internal bickering and jealousy issues are destroying practices, as well as opportunities to form a stronger base of political strength for the mental health segment. Other segments have their own unsavory position in the tug-of-war between state and federal government (bureaucrats vs. politicians) positioning. When wars break out, thousands lose their lives, but millions lose their internal and external sense of security.

THREATS TO AUTONOMY

The business side of practice brings to the table a number of hats. While a hard hat may protect your head from falling objects, your head is still vulnerable to heavy or sharp objects. In regards to a practice, there are things that you steel yourself against, but they can still affect you, such as hyperactive children, paranoid schizophrenias, and borderline personalities, as well as others. The crying and noise rings in one's head for hours after the office has been closed. These hats represent the tasks one accepts when accepting the opportunity to set up a practice, either individual or within a group. Tasks such as administrator, manager, entrepreneur, human resource manager, accounts payable, accounts receivable, clinician, educator, coach, community resource, filer, scheduler, sometimes as a grant writer, or even a missionary. Some of these tasks will be developed further in this chapter. The basic concept is that in private practice there are tasks to perform that are not reimbursable, and there are tasks that must be performed to protect the practice from audits, law suits, and claims against one's license(s). Detailed information published by insurance companies and state and federal agencies must be read due to the fact that it might eventually have a bearing on your practice. One thing I have learned is that representatives in state and federal legislatures frequently do not read the bills on which they are voting; astonishing news to constituents, but not to legislators. Secondly, unless a provider is prepared and willing to donate to re-election coffers, do not expect to be notified about legislation that is pending that might have negative consequences on the practice. Many legislators will be willing to share emails or phone calls, and working with their staff can be very helpful. Many of the consequences due to the changes in health care reform are negative, and this is largely due to poor communications between those who have the information and those who need the information. Businesses thrive on information. Corporations used to have seers, those who were thought to have supernatural powers to determine future political, economic, and business climates. Now the seers have doctorate degrees and write books about the art of planning for the future in a shaky global economy amid threats to our national security. Thus the underlining thrust of the homeland security industry and vendors, including professional organizations, offering credentials of memberships. In the years to come there might be positive benefits to the general population, as well as to providers, but that is yet to be realized. Issues that affect the autonomy of a practice allow the tail to control the direction of the dog. Providers are disturbed and confused by outsiders determining how their practice will be administered. One EAP social worker called and said that she didn't approve of the "robot message" on my answering machine and until it was changed, we would not receive any further referrals.

CONFLICTS WITH ADHD DISORDER BEING CALLED A DISABILITY

In most commerce activities there are examples of disbursement for no apparent reason other than an effort to garner more political strength within a block of voters. In health care one of these programs is awarding families who have a child(ren) who has been diagnosed with attention deficit disorder (ADD) or attention deficit hyperactivity disorder (ADHD) by giving the child(ren) a disability label plus a monthly income of $640 (SSI) plus, a home health care provider in some cases. More children in the U.S. are being diagnosed with ADHD than ever before—10.4 million in 2010—according to a new study that concluded a staggering rise in diagnoses of 66 percent since the year 2000 (Bindley, 2012, p. 1). This came from a research project of Craig Garfield, PhD, a researcher at Northwestern University and the lead author of the study. If the figure is only one million in 2010 that would mean that these children would be eligible in Texas to receive $7680 a year, or an estimated $7,680,000,000 for just one state! That is a lot of money to kids who are attending school, taking their medication, and doing the daily activities of other children their age. Medication and therapy help these children learn techniques to improve their concentration levels, which they can use the rest of their lives, thus improving their performance at school and/or on the job. States would love to keep this money, but no leader has stepped forward to suggest cutting the program. They are more likely to first ask doctors and therapists to accept a smaller reimbursement rate. This is a conflict with providers because they do not see ADD/ADHD as a disability.

CONFLICTS OF ROLES

The roles we take on within our practice range from healer and entrepreneur to educator and community resource. When HMOs say that Medicaid authorizes only three codes to bill: family, individual, and group, then how can you bill for educating and training parents to be better in their role as parents? When time is spent collaborating with a school counselor or PCP which code do you bill? These issues are similar to the confusion in therapy when a confrontation or a more subtle directive statement causes therapy to go in an unexpected direction. Not only are the codes outdated, but also the DSM-IV is nearing an end. The DSM-V looks promising, but the delivery is yet to be satisfactorily guaranteed. The purpose of such a therapeutic interaction justifies the use, but can also cause uncertainty, especially when your goal is to help the patient reach independent confidence in their decision making.

HEALER

The healer role stems from the missionary attitude that one knows a better way of life than another. If words, stories, metaphors, and suggestions lead to a reduction of symptoms, is one considered healed? If the definition of chronic pain is a pain that lasts for more than three months, then is the person cured if the symptoms do not return for three or more months? These are questions that can arise when discussing the length of treatment. Medicaid has a history of reimbursement for 30 treatment sessions in 12 months. With brief therapy and managed care has come the six sessions, which stop until the managed care gatekeeper receives further justification. If a case manager reviews your billings and sees a pattern of 20 plus sessions for 90% of your patients, they may flag your practice for an audit. Sometimes an audit means copying the files they've requested and sending them to their office, or they may send someone to visit your office to re-educate staff members.

EDUCATOR

The educator role occurs when you research material, and then print out information regarding a diagnosis, a disorder, or a series of parenting skill techniques for the patient, who might lack Internet access. This is likely to occur in rural and border communities, but may also occur in metropolitan communities where there is an education deficit population. One complaint of patients is that their PCP does not spend enough time listening to them; they frequently have more questions later and, if seen by a psychotherapist, it is not uncommon to have their questions brought to the sessions.

COMMUNITY RESOURCES

Community resources are of value to the PCPs, as well as to the families of patients. Knowing there are specialists in other cities that could see them can be beneficial to patients as to the direction of therapy, as well as the outcome. The ability to refer patients to a source who can help them obtain food stamps, temporary shelter, or babysitting services while the parents work are all important to therapy success. Understanding Maslow's Hierarchy of Needs helps document the value of the session, including the referral. Some-times a therapist can feel as though they are being used to document a disorder, such as ADD/ADHD, in order for the government to pay a monthly disability check. Once they get the check the family isn't seen again, unless the child is suspended from school for fighting. At that time an evaluation would be performed to assess the presenting problem, along with the onset of problems, what treatment, if any, has been offered, and how successful that has been. What is often discovered is that the child is no longer taking the medication and it's been at least two years since a mental health provider saw them. Having a letter of non-compliance in the child's records alerts the PCP; however, the state may never know and so the family continues to receive Medicaid, as well as disability income. These issues are a cause of alarm and concern for therapists who believe in the value of their treatment. The question to be answered is: do therapists have an ethical or legal obligation to call the Attorney General, whose department supervises these types of services?

ENTREPRENEUR

The role of entrepreneur leads to repeated conflicts with clinical issues. An entrepreneur invests in a company or business for the purpose of making a profit. Clinicians could agree on the first part of this sentence; the latter part is denied unless the word salary is substituted for the word profit. In the business world profit is not naturally associated with salary. A salary is part of the operating expenses and covers employees as well as the owner. After all overhead expenses are paid, the money left over can be attributed to profit or to a future investment project, such as replacing the roof of the building; therefore, the future endeavor would be considered part of the operating expenses and not a profit.

A therapist or physician in private practice is an entrepreneur who is tasked with many different jobs. Human resource management presents a number of issues that can cripple a practice, such as not having the time or resources to check references, or to do a drug test, or to check criminal records. For example, unbeknownst to me, a secretary I hired was on probation for welfare fraud. I eventually found out after he was arrested and needed to make bail after not making a payment to the court. Another one of my employees signed the employee contract as a licensed professional counselor, then stole files from the office and eventually sued me for not paying him enough.

When employees quit they often try to argue that you did something unethical or illegal and then threaten to use their local resources to fight for their "unemployment rights" even when they've failed to meet employee standards. Every employee that receives worker's compensation can run your tax rate for the unemployment fund higher, which adds more expenses and decreases the amount of funds available to pay. I know of one psychologist that couldn't cash her payroll checks for seven months, had to close her office, and eventually accepted a position in a university hospital institution.

Business often requires having more than one bank account, i.e., personal, corporate or business, and sometimes an account designated for end of year taxes. When writing a business plan and developing a three-year projection, it helps if you consult the local Small Business Administration (SBA), which has expertise in formatting such a plan. They can offer a clearer picture of what bankers and loan officers want to see in a projection. Spending time with these people can be worthwhile in a number of ways including learning the language of loan officers, and understanding where there are weaknesses in the plan, and how it is presented on paper.

DEFENSIVE PRACTICE

In a one-person office the provider is the one that develops the programs offered to patients and PCPs, establishes testing or evaluation surveys and initial assessment forms, as well as other forms, and puts into place an annual internal audit system. Compliance and practice policy manuals are office essentials. Such policies may cover how the therapist determines the levels of anxiety, depression, or ADD/ADHD. The more defensive tasks that are incorporated, the less time for therapy, and there will be fewer billings, which translates into less weekly or monthly reimbursement checks.

Defensive practice means anticipation of audits, investigations, and complaints to the licensing boards. While there is no fireproof policy that will prevent these three demons of destruction, there are some things a provider or practice manager can do in preparation for such events:

- Develop a compliance manual. Group practices are likely to have a compliance team that meets monthly and keeps notes of their meetings in a folder or binder which documents compliance attempts.
- Hold annual audits of your files.
- Include documentation of dismissal/termination of employees in the compliance manual.
- Develop a policy and procedures manual that includes policies in regards to billing, collections, chain-of-command, policies on documentation, employee contracts (in a small office), and procedures for correcting billing errors or files with inadequate documentation (from an annual internal audit). Create a company policy on hiring a contract auditor for potentially inappropriate billing or when an employee is terminated and issues of impropriety are suggested. Most corporate attorneys will ask that they be the ones hiring the outside auditor for the corporation, due to issues of confidentiality.
- Read bulletins from MCOs, HMOs, Medicaid, and Medicare. Keep them in a binder and review them annually. Check the licensing board website annually for new rulings, changes in policy or recommendations.
- Keep a binder for all corporate attorney correspondence.
- Keep binders for all S&Rs (billing information).
- Keep a binder of all CEUs and training of staff internally.
- Consult with your corporate attorney on a regular basis.
- Consult with a specialist on legislative changes that might affect your practice.

MANAGER

The dilemma of having to constantly choose between clinical tasks and business tasks is ongoing and often unrewarding. Determining priorities is part of management tasks:

- Management of human resources
- Management of accounts payable and receivable

- Management of duties of staff
- Management of time
- Management of planning for CEUs
- Business trips to professional association board meetings and professional association conferences
- Ensuring maintenance for cleaning the office
- Having resources to make office repairs
- Management of security issues of the office (i.e., how to handle an angry person who walks into the office and disrupts a session as well as upsets the families waiting in the reception room).

Each project has a timeline and clinicians have to operate between certain hours, during which time they have scheduled patient sessions, return phone calls, write letters, and perhaps have a coffee break, or maybe even lunch. People in the field for several years understand that business is carried home frequently, and when they have a family to care for and nourish, their own physical and emotional energy is drained.

Managing an office is a tedious job and requires time and energy dedicated to a variety of tasks. It is very demanding as there are so many tasks within any health care office or clinic. The manager should be someone with a business background in health care management. They need to know about the problems of billing and collections and how to best handle problems that arise from panels who demand more accreditation information for licensing the practice. Every hour that a licensed health care provider is involved with a business question or an issue, is an hour lost from producing revenue and this is more frustrating to the provider than dealing with a difficult medical or mental health problem.

While time management has been discussed, as well as the value of understanding and working with budget worksheets, there is a less colorful and more mundane task that can be a stumbling block to time management success: paperwork. It is not uncommon for providers of all disciplines to have stacks of homework, which includes letters to write, calls to return, and material to research (articles on disorders, diseases, and mind/body relationship issues and treatment, etc.). Books get pulled out and need to be replaced in the bookcase. Messages and calls to return need to be addressed at the end of the day prior to leaving the office. Having a staff member who is not afraid of detail work and can file correctly is an asset and can be hard to find in rural and border communities. Problems can arise from failure to keep on top of this work and can mean lost time in searching for files, forms, and messages. In addition, USBs used in transferring data from one computer to another can, due to their size, be easily lost, stolen, or placed with a patient file. Having a backup system for a USB will reduce the loss when it is mishandled or stolen and you are looking for a letter or other stored material.

Having the backup on a separate PC that is not connected to the Internet can create a safe harbor. Another helpful tip is to download files from the working PC or laptop to a disc once a week and then store the disk in a locked cabinet.

The question of billing and collections is a three-pronged problem:

- Qualified billers are extremely difficult to find in rural and border communities
- Outsourcing billing costs are 8%-14% per collection
- A qualified biller handles all problems of collections and billings, including keeping up with all new laws and changes in reimbursement rates, as well as other restrictions for billings and collections.

MCOs and HMOs are required to send letters to the patient, as well as the provider, on any rejections of claims. There are cases where they have failed to send providers vital and timely information, and due to this oversight providers continued seeing patients who have been told that they had not met the deductible for the year and as a result, the patient had to pay the balance. In many cases this led to patients refusing to pay, they stopped coming in when asked for the money, and the provider was left with an unpaid bill. Add four or five of these cases and one can see the provider losing a lot of money due to the lack of adequate and timely information being shared by the MCO or HMO. There is also less costly software billing programs available for therapists for in-house billing. The cost of not having an experienced biller with knowledge of the verification process, how to bill different MCOs and HMOs, and how to solve billing errors can lead to greater losses. Most therapists are reluctant to send people to credit bureaus and collection agencies and as a result, that means losing additional money each year.

Uniting the independent therapist, psychologist, or social worker with a network of providers, or a group of providers that unite to ensure compliance with current rules and regulations of CHS and HMOs, including Medicare and Medicaid, is very important. With this network, providers will have the training needed to access initial and follow-up testing software, documentation procedures, referral hardware and software, and a billing company that has experience with the current rules and regulations.

EXPERT WITNESS

This position is not a very comfortable role to play, as none of us are "experts" by some definitions, while everyone has an "expertise" in something. Court cases often require a mental health physician to provide expert testimony for cases such as child abuse or neglect, child custody cases, trauma cases (accidents, victim position), and sexual offender cases. The more rural your practice, the more likely the provider has had the victim as a patient. In a metropolitan community many psychologists refuse to see cases where there may be a need for an expert witness, while there are a number of psychologists that search out cases where they can provide testimony. The more providers train for presenting testimony, the better prepared they are and the more likely they will be accepted by the court. It is a risky business in that the defense will search into your background for things that they may use to discredit your testimony. Sometimes you can be expected to be in the courtroom for several hours, as the attorney suspending your testimony will have you there early to go over questions and ask for any new developments in the case.

FILE STORAGE: RISKS AND LIABILITIES

Insurance companies and Medicaid and Medicare require that files be kept for at least 10 years after one leaves practice. Some may require that children's files be kept until their 25th birthday. The storage for these files needs to be reasonably secure. Having them in locked file cabinets behind a locked door, or in a locked storage compartment is more than likely going to be adequate. It may not be required to be in a locked file cabinet if it is in a locked storage compartment since many file cabinet locks deteriorate over time. If storage compartments run an average of $80 a month for ten years that would equate to about $1000 per year or $10,000 over 10 years. If a business is sold then the files can be transferred to the new owner. In any case this can be precarious, as people have been known to cut the locks off of storage compartments, and if the file cabinet is not locked, or if the files are in boxes, there could be exposure to the elements. Even if you are not held liable, you could be seriously embarrassed. Consult with your attorney for the best way to handle not only the files, but also all paperwork regarding billings, collections, forms, and books from the insurance companies for the previous ten years.

COLLABORATIVE PARTNERS

This refers to the requirements of insurers, including Medicaid and Medicare, that providers have a multi-disciplinary group or that the physicians collaborate with mental health providers and social workers, as is appropriate. This means that each doctor and each allied provider have the hardware and software that protects confidentiality as outlined by the federal government and this can cost from several thousands of dollars to over $30,000. Normally this equipment and software will place a date and time on each transaction so that if there is a breakdown, an auditor can determine who failed the system. Each provider that collaborates with an ACO or a CCO has the possibility of contributing to the bonus program for the group that has their money invested in the organization. If the organization saves money, the members receive a bonus. If there are no savings, their reimbursement rate may decline.

This chapter has presented some important points, including:

- Over the past 40 years the business of therapy has taken form and with it, another branch has been growing: the political side of therapy, although not at the same growth rate of knowledge and appreciation of value. Providers are slow in understanding these two growth areas. Just when we think we may have a handle on it, another segment or branch springs forth. For most providers, if the business side of practice was an awkward pill to take, the fact that politics and corporate America are working hand-in-hand with the government to encourage cost savings will be an even more difficult pill to swallow.
- Positioning within the health care system continues to gain in stature with the Accountability Act. While this is not a new relationship for many providers, it will force those who have held back to finally see the light and find groups to join in order to survive the latest reforms.
- The Achilles heel of mental health providers was discussed with the hope that more providers will find ways to support unification efforts to strengthen our base of existence within the health care industry. By becoming more active in professional associations, a leader within the community is willing to share their time with PTAs and church groups to educate parents and others about the changes facing primary care physicians and mental health providers. Leadership is necessary because a leader shares their values and talents with others. The general population needs to learn about their role within modern health care: an informed patient who takes responsibility for staying healthy.
- The different hats of responsibility were offered as a way to introduce the different tasks of a practice, which underlines the lack of time, energy, and revenues to complete all the tasks solo. It also explains why many are not making enough money to justify their sacrifices as well as their educational and business investments in private practice, and this reinforces the joining or forming of groups of interdisciplinary health care providers within a community.

Chapter Five

Creating a Value Added Service

Value is the quality of importance that one places on a product or service at a certain point of cost, or time, or availability. Fast food restaurants see convenience and speed of service as increasing value. In other words, more people will choose to eat at a fast food restaurant more for the convenience and speed of service than for menu choices and quality of food. Car dealers sell through advertisements and media ads the ease of purchase: "just sign your name and the car is yours;" or "credit is no problem;" or "we have the lowest financing rates;" and "we have many colors and models to choose from." Educational institutions are selling education with distance learning and Internet courses with government financing. Banks are offering low interest rates but not for people who want to build. Banks normally make a loan and keep the paper for one year and then sell it to a mortgage company. Today these mortgage companies are not buying loan paper as in the past, given the crisis created when many mortgage companies bought worthless loan paper that was bound to fail when the economy changed. Primary care physicians normally do not advertise, but people go to them when they are sick or need some prevention treatment or evaluation. Why should anyone see a psychotherapist?

Health is value to the individual and family but not as much as when good health is lost from an accident, disease, or disorder. Ask an individual who has developed juvenile diabetes what this health problem has done to his/her health as well as daily activities. What about their dreams for their future? Or the soldier returning from war with no legs? Or the family whose father has had a stroke and may never be able to work again. What is the value of good health to these and other cases like them? What is the value of a good education without the resources to obtain it? What is the value of good mental health to someone who is suffering from major depression with suicidal ideations? It comes down to the point where the individual chooses to stop feeling so bad. For years people have chosen not to go to dentists because of the pain. Today, dentists are reviving their practices with procedures that are less painful, offering medication for the pain, and offering the equivalent of a facelift with a complete change in the appearance of the teeth. Psychotherapists have moved from behind the patient to sitting across from the patient and encouraging an interaction rather than just having the patient talk without the interaction. Like the dentists, psychotherapists have had to learn ways to reduce the pain of therapy. One way is to collaborate with the patient's PCP or to refer them to a psychiatrist. As the shortage of psychiatrists has increased, the job of medication is falling on the shoulders of PCPs.

When discussing the value of health care, one course is to ask what about the worth of your life. One way to evaluate the worth of one's life is to ask someone to perform risky jobs for money. Looking back to European battles, kings who offered land and/or a share of the spoils of battle were able to recruit more soldiers. When the king reneged on the agreement the warriors turned against the king. Soldiers often sign up for a tour in the military out of a sense of patriotism, like the period of time immediately after the Twin Towers in New York were destroyed and the Pentagon was attacked. In between crises people tend to take their time to think before signing up at a recruiter's office. Those that are motivated to sign up do it for the educational benefits and/or for a job. A soldier risking their life in the Middle East because they need money for college and they need a job are implicitly stating: my life is worth $40,000 a year (salary) and the chance to use the educational benefits ($100,000). Therefore, using these figures and the length of term (4 years) the value of their life is $260,000. Economists and researchers that have studied death risks by occupation and industry have concluded that a statistical life is worth between $4.7 million to $8.5 million. These values account for the influence of clustering of the job risk variable and compensating differentials for both workers' compensation and nonfatal job risks (Viscusi, 2004).

Costs of medical technology has increased health care costs more than an office visit to one's primary care provider, or a few psychotherapy sessions, or speech therapy for children. However, the benefits from each unit of an MRI or one brain scan can be significantly more valuable on the side of the scans if they find an organic cause of suffering. Still, employers are balking at paying increased premiums and taxpayers are screaming about rising tax rates for property.

> The question is not whether we should take on the challenge of putting a price on life, but how we should do it. Economists, health services researchers, and public health officials have advocated a variety of approaches. Depending on

the methodology, the value of a life ranges from less than $200,000 to $5 million or more. Smaller values are based on methods that ignore or minimize the intrinsic value of life. But surveys and evidence from real-world behavior confirm that most people hold their lives dear and place a very high value on the intrinsic value (Dranove, 2003, p.159-160).

Employers base the life of employees on the value of their work to the company. While the value on a sheet metal worker may be $90,000 a year (what each worker's production can mean to the company revenues), to the CEO whose worth is the value of his or her decision-making skills, contacts with important businesses in their industry, or those contacts in Congress who have a great deal of influence when selling to the government. The costs of replacing a worker on the lower level of the decision making system is less than the cost of finding a replacement for the CEOs, in other words, there are more sheet metal workers than CEOs in the construction industry. Comparing values of health to the sports world where the individual's health is paramount to performance, and the replacement can be equally costly, not only in dollars but in wins and losses of games. If a truck driver has emotional problems and chooses not to seek a remedy for that pain, the results may be catastrophic if there is an accident. For many it is a trade-off between the inconvenience of taking time from school or work to spend an hour with a therapist to talk about difficult problems and feelings. For some it is like adding pain to stop the original pain. We can stop a tooth ache by smashing our finger in the door. We haven't stopped the pain but we have temporarily replaced it with a larger pain. Some people replace depression with cocaine but when the effects of cocaine fade, the old pain of depression remains.

SELF CARE

Job burnout is a popular term used when derivatization turns tension and energy into mush. One possible reason for this chemical transformation is the inner core of the provider where the basic belief resides that states they do not have the right to have their own needs met; that their only pathway to a reward is in giving up of one's self and serving others. Therapists are often more absorbed in the lives of others and lose focus of their own deficits. It goes back to the religious training of "it's better to give than to receive." In a spiritual sense one is building stars for their crown when they go to heaven. This self-denying comes with many inner conflicts that is observable when watching how they spend more time with patients than with family members, more time working and less time making money; which may explain why therapists are often very poor managers of money. Self-care is the process that focuses on developing a healthy self-respect and an awareness of self-worth (Bernhard, 1975).

Most self-help books would suggest that a person with symptoms of job burnout find something else to do, like going walking or jogging, swim, listen to music that softens your tension, and consider changing jobs. One self-help audio tape shares this bit of wisdom:

> Burnout brings with it many losses, which can often go unrecognized. Unrecognized losses trap a lot of your energy. It takes a tremendous amount of emotional control to keep yourself from feeling the pain of these losses. When you recognize these losses and allow yourself to grieve them, you release that trapped energy and open yourself to healing.

- Loss of the idealism or dream with which you entered your career
- Loss of the role or identity that originally came with your job
- Loss of physical and emotional energy
- Loss of friends, fun, and sense of community
- Loss of esteem, self-worth, and sense of control and mastery
- Loss of joy, meaning and purpose that make work—and life—worthwhile (Luban, 1994)

Another source offers a difference between stress and burnout. While we need stress to stand up, walk, eat, and work, stress can reach a breakpoint and that point is called a state of too much stress, or burnout:

> Burnout is a state of emotional, mental, and physical exhaustion caused by excessive and prolonged stress. It occurs when you feel overwhelmed and unable to meet constant demands. As the stress continues, you begin to lose the interest or motivation that led you to take on a certain role in the first place. Burnout reduces your productivity and saps your energy, leaving you feeling increasingly helpless, hopeless, cynical, and resentful. Eventually, you may feel like you have nothing more to give. Burnout, on the other hand, is about not enough. Being burned out means feeling empty, devoid of motivation, and beyond caring. People experiencing burnout often don't see any hope of positive change in their situations. If excessive stress is like drowning in responsibilities, burnout is being all dried up. One other difference between stress and burnout: While you're usually aware of being under a lot of stress, you don't always notice burnout when it happens (Smith, Segal, and Segal, 2012).

One of the symptoms of depression, in addition to those offered above, is personal hygiene. In Texas Fridays are historically blue jeans days worn with a white dress shirt. Wearing jeans everyday would be careless and signal an "I don't care attitude," or "what difference does it make, anyway?" Nick Cummings, PhD, pioneer in starting graduate schools in psychology that include business courses, a former president of American Psychological Association, and the Chairman of the Cummings Foundation, argues that we providers should dress like professionals all the time (Thomas, Cummings, O'Donahue, 2002). Some might argue that would be good advice for those working in hospitals and corporations, but those in private practice in rural and border communities normally dress according to local cultural traditions. One therapist noted that when he wore a dress shirt, matching tie, and sport coat there have been not a few comical remarks about his appearance. He works in the rural community near the border with Mexico. Two people offered the question, "What are you doing? Trying to show off to us?" Therefore, I have returned to the dress shirt and slacks and an occasional sport coat, but no tie, except when I am testifying in court. Then court etiquette demands it (professional etiquette) including polished shoes.

Compassion fatigue is another term for burnout when applied to the helping professionals. It refers to a physical, emotional, and spiritual fatigue or exhaustion that is viewed as a one-way street, where providers give a great deal of energy and compassion to others over a period of time, yet do not receive enough compassion or reassurance from others in the field due to isolation, working in rural or border communities where there are not very many colleagues to ventilate or mentor. It is this constant giving process that can lead to depression, a loss of sight of the mission, and a loss of energy to keep fighting back against reimbursement cutbacks and other legislation or regulations that reduce the practice of mental health. In addition, administrative and law enforcement bureaucrats force audits and audit results without any hope of appeals. It is as if they say, "fight it if you can, but we will prevail no matter what." Such an attitude, real or distorted, is prevalent in the business of health care. As a result providers have lost trust in their professional associations, in the licensing boards, and in managed care corporations.

WHAT IS THE VALUE OF PSYCHOTHERAPY?

Psychotherapists utilize talk therapy to encourage a patient to change their perceptions, their thoughts, and their behaviors in order to accomplish what the patient deems as important in their lives such as improving the quality of their lives. Each therapy session is different from others because the people sitting across from the therapist are unique, and their problems which may seem similar to others, are unique to them. Basic theory of human nature may suggest that all people are born evil, or that we are all born with a perfect body, but as we grow and develop, we develop bad habits, learn bad words, feel bad pain, think bad thoughts, and behave badly. Are we then inherently evil? Theologians might argue that we are perfect until we are born and then are born into sin. Evil is sin, and emotional and physical pain may not be a sin but a consequence of a sin or a bad habit (alcoholism, drug abuse, and other unhealthy life styles). In therapy people are encouraged to ventilate their feelings, good and bad, and to decrease their frustration and fears.

Therapists offer encouragement for patients to grow into healthy, happy, people who can be as productive as they choose to be. The essential core of a person is often suppressed or denied, and anxiety, depression, and fears overcome the positive aspects of one's inner nature. Religious leaders will talk about the weakness of our nature and that a closer relationship with God can be helpful as the person struggles with the evil side of life and life choices. Psychologists and psychotherapists observe people and they listen, something that is lacking within the medical model of healing. Studying others can teach us about mistakes and shortcomings, about consequences and choices, and about the fragilities of life and the power of human passion and determination to overcome obstacles. One of the basic points we have learned is that every act that destroys our neurons, every act of evil that is recorded in our subconsciouness makes us despise ourselves and is self-destructive. Teaching these key points to patients as part of therapy can open windows of opportunity to view a different pathway that can lead to the mountain top or a higher point of inner tranquility and balance.

> Psychotherapy remains the ally of self preservation, self, and self care. It teaches us to value our minds as our most important resource because the mind is the powerhouse that generates ideas, makes decisions, and funds power for action. When we acquire access to this resource, we are able to move our intentions out of our minds and into the world. From its inception through the present, the fundamental purpose of psychotherapy remains to strengthen the mind, the psyche, and the soul. In the valuing of our words, talk therapy teaches us the value of taking ourselves seriously—finally placing value where it belongs (Frost, 2012).

The relationship between the mind and body in the healing process is built into many courses in psychology and psychotherapy. There are many good reasons while this relationship has become a more valid and reliable basis to form therapeutic relationships. Beginning with the work of biofeedback we learned new ways to monitor and change muscular signals and brain signals through instant feedback.

> As a medical tool, biofeedback is used to treat specific malfunctioning systems such as fecal incontinence; as a relaxation technique to release stress within a homeostatic balance; as a research tool to investigate functional dynamics of the organism. In this process, feedback enhances the autonomy of the individual. Feedback points out that we are so often reacting instead of acting, responding instead of initiating. Now we can learn strategies to help us change our behaviors. Feedback allows us to become synchronous with our own bio-psychological needs. In fact, health occurs when mind/body/spirit are in synchrony. (Peper, Ancoli, and Quinn, 1983, p. 563).

Hypnosis is more prevalent then biofeedback in psychotherapy offices because it does not require expensive hardware and software. It is very useful in teaching patients to regain self-regulation, reducing negative effects of stress, and empowering the individual to practice the same techniques in their own homes. Milton Erickson was a pioneer in the modern development of hypnosis in the offices of therapists. He bridged the gap between hypnosis and other psychotherapies.

> Hypnotic phenomena occur as the result of communication and concentrated internal attention, not from some physical difference between the normal waking state and trance states. Biofeedback studies of EEG and oxygen consumption during meditation, sleep, hypnotic trance, and waking reveal that the hypnotic state is most similar to the waking state. In other words, the physiological phenomena produced by communication and internal search process are most like those of the normal waking state. It follows that communication in psychotherapy and other waking states produces and uses trance phenomena under various guises (Lankton, Stephen Ryan, 1982, p. 142).

Words used to create change in psychotherapy are similar to words used in hypnosis. The inductions into an altered state of consciousness and some goals are different than a typical psychotherapy session. Both use words to educate, train, encourage insightful work, and to encourage a reduction of illogical thoughts and feelings and to change the physiology relationships and brain functions to reduce fears, anxiety, pain, and despair. Psychotherapy is the bridging of the gap between therapist and patient to transfer information that can change feelings and thoughts that allows the patient to regain a sense of inner balance and personal satisfaction in their lives.

> Deepak Chopra, an endocrinologist who has synthesized ancient and modern medicine, physics, and philosophy, teaches that mental awareness results in physical chemistry—and that our reality is a result of our perceptions. His is a world of *infinite possibilities*. Physician Larry Dossey argues that the emotional and mental currency of *meaning* actually enters the body and alters its cells. His provocative research on the power of prayer has led to large-scale studies that are influencing the direction of medicine. Medical psychologist Joan Borysenko demonstrates how the mind, body, and spirit are inseparably linked— and are at work in the intricacies of human immunity (Karrebm, Hafen, Smith, Frandsen, 2006, p. xv).

> As more and more research findings are reported the gap between the body and mind has disappeared. The pain is not only in the head but in all parts of the body. Psychotherapists for decades have been talking about this connection because they can observe and hear the pathways. A more recent study describes the value of emotional awareness of pain. The medical model of identifying underlying causes of pain and discomfort has been to look for structural damage (tissues, muscular, skeletal). Physicians are now acknowledging that

many pain syndromes have psychophysiologic foundations. There is evidence to support the theory that genetic predispositions reside in our tissue and neurons, and there are studies that show how they can be triggered to activate (Caspi, Sugden, Moffitt, 2003) and a study to show how they can be controlled and not activated (Taylor, 2010).

Pain can originate in the absence of a tissue disorder in the area where pain is being felt, as seen in phantom limb syndrome. A study by Derbyshire et al confirmed that pain initiated by the brain is identical to pain originating in peripheral tissue (Schubiner and Betzold, 2012, p. 1).

Schubiner points out that there is a psychology to pain and most of our thoughts and emotions originate in our subconscious. The subconscious is where emotional threats are first noticed and then sends out sensations that notify the parts of our physical body that needs to be on alert. Such physical reactions can cause gastrointestinal symptoms, headaches, lower back and neck pain, and other symptoms. Those with history of childhood illnesses, injuries, or abuse may experience these symptoms sooner than others and the symptoms might last longer than for others without that history. Later in life the pain may be diagnosed as fibromyalgia, peptic ulcers, or abdominal or pelvic pain. Schubiner argues that these disorders and symptoms may be traced to recent efforts to avoid a hostile situation, family violence, or an angry employer. He notes that these people tend to have a highly developed conscience. Internal pain, such as the result of family violence or childhood abuse, can be trapped by suppression of emotions and may lead to chronic pain pathways.

Schubiner concludes that:

- Not all practitioners are trained to conduct an in-depth psychological interview beginning with childhood history and possible psychological factors that could create psychophysiologic disorders.
- Though family histories are seldom seen, they can be critical in ferreting out a history of abuse: emotional, physical, and sexual.
- History of bullying can be an important ingredient in present day reactions.
- History of patterns of resentment, losses, abandonment, fearful events, and feelings of guilt.
- Initial interviews often include history but not all focus on the above factors. Triggers are events, relationships, a certain smell, or imagery, or words interpreted as a threat.
- Stressful childhood events play powerful roles in the development of psychophysiologic disorders.
- Successfully treated patients are those who are convinced that they have PPD rather than a structural disease process and that they have the re-

sources to overcome the obstacles to the pain, and are willing to devote the time needed to learn the steps to overcoming PPD.
- The practitioner's job is to help patients develop the first of these attributes; the rest is up to the patient (Schubiner and Betzold, 2012, pp.4-7).

Practitioners have many pioneers in the field of medicine and mental health to thank for breaking ground for further advancement of the theories and treatment techniques but also for sharing the value of their profession to health care industry administers, political leaders, and to the general public. Anything we can do to promote the welfare of our profession adds value to our services. Collaboration requires that we share the wealth of knowledge that is growing each year through experience, research, published articles, and books, and at national conventions. It is an obligation that is being compromised by the turf wars between disciplines, the lack of leadership in graduate schools, and the tendency for providers not to become active in politics. It is also damaged by the tendency for many providers to withdraw from the process by not being active for their profession, or not attending professional association conferences, or *dropping out* and losing hope.

As the value of lower rates affects corporations, the theory is that corporations will pass on their savings in lower care prices, or lower food prices, etc. But there is no guarantee. The employer can pocket the savings and the employees will pay the price by paying higher co-payments, being denied certain services that were once offered, and losing accessibility. As the cost cuts fall down the ladder, they end up in the offices of physicians and psychotherapists. Mental health offices are closing, physicians are retiring early, and patients are having problems finding the services that were offered in their community prior to the reform changes. A neurologist closed his office to open up a school. A psychologist closed her office to pursue interior decorating, which she had started as hobby. A psychotherapist closed his office to work in a non-profit organization. A social worker closed his office to return to law school. A psychiatrist closed her office to teach in a graduate school.

If grants continue to decrease, non-profits will not be able to fill the gap. State grants to community mental health organizations have been recipients of cuts in funding and they pass this down to the consumer in the form of fewer services or less services from licensed professionals. This amounts to less accessibility to quality providers who have years of experience who are now replaced, by necessity, by less qualified providers (less education, not licensed by the state, and with fewer formal and informal training experiences). The rational is: "Everyone has to share the costs so everyone can have some health care benefits." Pharmacies may be going out of business because their profit margin is being cut by lower reimbursement for filling prescriptions for Medicaid patients. Those pharmacies that have catered to the Medicaid population for years will be the hardest hit. Since many of them are in lower-income locations, such as rural and border states, they may be forced to shut their stores and people Medicaid patients will have to go further into town, travel to a larger city who would have a chain of stories who offer pharmacy services in order to get their prescriptions filled. Some may resort to going into Mexico to purchase medication, which has been an option for years. In two short years a tidal wave of newly insured patients will be enrolled and will be asking for benefits they have been denied in the past. This is scaring the politicians and the budget administrators (government and insurance companies) who will be dealt a problem that has only been tested in theory studies scenario research.

For the value of mental health services to be experienced it must be shared. If the current structure will not accommodate mental health services, we must find a way. There is potential for mental health to grow within the ACOs and COOs, but a lot of people need help from a lot more providers to make this happen. We need to find a voice and a medium to be heard and leaders to encourage a new pathway that is encompassing and not exclusionary.

CAREER BUILDING

Private practitioners tend to practice with a narrow focus. For decades they have focused on issues of ethical practice and clinical proficiencies. Then came the issue of the business of therapy that one psychologist wrote about in his book, underlining the lack of knowledge of the management and business side of health care practices by psychologists and psychotherapists (Pressman, 1979, p. vii). The same remains today as physicians and therapists are trying to catch up with the business side of practice. As they have done so, time has to be taken from direct contact with patients that are the primary source of revenues. Since time is money, dedicating time for career building seems a bit self-destructive. This is due to a loss of appreciation for opportunities that can advance careers in more than one way. By becoming stationary we lose opportunities to improve our profession. We need to build care pathways not only to help individuals but the profession.

They are so focused on protecting one's practice, in building up referral sources, and in doing all the tasks that one in private practice has to do that providers neglect the updating of a quality curriculum vitae. After 10 years in private practice a provider can forget all the tasks that he/she is responsible for, and when they start looking at job tasks on websites they can become frustrated and intimidated by all the professionally written duties required of a position. It is very common for providers in private practice to work 70 plus hours a week. Many providers have worked six days a week and tackle paperwork on Sundays before the football games begin.

Some providers, like psychologist Lynn Friedman, develop subspecialties that can attract people with different needs. She also offers career counseling and places a map to her office on her website: http://www.washington-dc-psychologist.com/private-practice.html. Others work within organizations and specialize in organizational development, human resources, career assessments, and developing programs addressing issues of employees and their families. Along the way they develop relationships with headhunters and use a skilled resume builder to advertise their accomplishments and attract new offers of employment opportunities.

Part of self care is coming to the realization that being a workaholic is not an asset, it is a liability. If workaholics do not change their work schedules or their careers, the body will do it for them. Build up a relationship with a professional resume/vitae writer and a headhunter that knows the field and begin grooming for a new career if you fit this mold. Writing a resume or vitae is a growing art, as is the preparation for an interview. There are consultants making large amounts of money training professionals how to write about their experiences and what to leave out. They will discuss the cover letter and the key factors of an interview. Providers often seem reluctant to learn this new phase of career development, but success can mean doubling one's income or being pushed aside by an advancing current of change.

PROFESSIONAL ASSOCIATIONS

The ineffectiveness of professional associations to unify, in order to strengthen their bargaining powers, has failed the profession. A reasonable person could expect greater effort from the American Medical Association (AMA), the State Association of Medical Providers, the American Psychological Association (APA), the National Social Work Association (NSWA), the American Chiropractic Association (ACA), the American Counselors Association (ACA), the American Physical Therapy Association (APTA), the American Psychotherapy Association (APA), the American Psychiatric Association (APA), the American Mental Health Association (AMHA), American Marriage and Family Therapists (AMFT), American Nurses Association (ANA), American Respiratory Therapist Association (ARTA), National Association of Professional Psychology Providers (NAPPP), and the National Academy of Practice (NA). These professional associations have shown no ability or desire to organize anyone but their closest associates to oppose changes that affect their membership. They have acted as if their members want warm fuzzies, continuing education courses, and the latest in research or application. The numbers of medical doctors has been estimated to be near 800,000 while not all are members of the AMA, some choosing to support their state association instead of the national organization. The APA has a membership around 100,000 and the NAPPP has another 25, 000. That leaves about 400,000 nurses, 200,000 master level counselors and therapists, and 400,000 social workers. No matter what the exact numbers, they still add up to over a million providers who are unrepresented or underrepresented in the political arena. Corporate America has the money and resources to out fight any efforts of providers to try to get a stronger voice in Washington. If states can close down unions, then what can a small group of providers expect to accomplish? The nationalization is created out of the authority of the highest political levels in state and federal governments. One can argue that it is just a political debate; but it is more than just a disagreement or a debate of economics. The real power to control practices and lives is being practiced in corporate America as you read this book. It is also being planned in state and federal governmental agencies by bureaucrats and elected officials. Why are they doing all the talking? Why are we not part of the discussion and change process?

IS HEALTH CARE A RIGHT?

This is a question that has been debated in the past two or three decades and will continue to be on agenda for the next decade. The conference rooms are filled by legislators, health care administrators, and researchers, as well as the general public. It is not going away just because the current mood is to argue about doing away or cutting back entitlement programs. There are so many hysterical fears and drama on both sides of the argument for health care coverage for everyone. The second factor is moving from multiple payers to a single payer system. Considering health care as a *right* is at the base of all of these questions about health care costs, accessibility, and financing. This is the cutting line for the haves and the have nots. Each has interesting points that need to be discussed, but they are both biased positions and neither side is listening to the other. In between them are the providers (medical and mental health) who are committed to service but do not believe they should be forced to live in poverty. Even missionaries and preachers get paid; some evangelists are multi-millionaires.

If any of these questions sound familiar, then you are old enough to remember the debate over the 1964 Civil Rights Act. Like yesteryear the argument was that the government was overreaching their power and attempting to regulate commerce. The leaders of yesteryear included Senator Strom Thurmond, a Democrat from South Carolina, who denounced the Civil Rights Act as unconstitutional and beyond the realm of reason. He was outdated and there are Congress members who are outdated today. With the Supreme Court involvement in the discussion of health care reform, this marks another round of arguments against and for the Affordable Care Act that has the potential of going down to lower courts and into Congress committee rooms and then back up to the Supreme Court again. The argument that government does not need to be involved in regulating health care sounds like the arguments of the 1960s that argued "everyone has civil rights, it's just that some have more than others."

> The federal government is already deeply involved in regulating healthcare, not just through Medicare and Medicaid but also through a variety of regulations covering private plans—such as COBRA, which provides continued coverage for employees who leave a job. Much existing federal regulation of health coverage seeks to control the tens of billions of dollars a year that uninsured patients cost the system—costs we all pay through taxes and our own higher insurance premiums. The Affordable Care Act is simply another way of doing what the government already does. It makes sound financial sense to make sure everyone has insurance, because one way or another we end up paying for those who don't (Saporta, 2012).

COACHING

This is a spin-off from the field of counseling and psychotherapy. We may feel, at times, that we are the cheerleaders for our patients who are struggling with learning new techniques of relationship or personal growth. Our techniques are to assist people to learn new coping skills that can build meaningful relationships and to improve one's self-esteem. We do not advertise that we can solve problems but problem solving techniques are used to assist the patient to overcome their fears, anxieties, and reluctance to make the choices needed that can bring resolutions to their conflicts. The advertised field of coaching is very similar but they normally do not advertise that they are therapists, as that might misrepresent their services and the fact that they are not licensed to practice psychotherapy or to bill insurances.

In many of the training programs it is not unusual to find the literature referring to a professional coaching organization that sets *rules and regulations*. Advertisements for training may state that their training certifications are *credible around the world*. One coaching institute has created a curriculum made up of two components: core curriculum and certification program. The core curriculum includes:

- Fundamentals: The section sounds like the trainer listens to experiences of the trainee and provides some feedback.

- Fulfillment: This section provides information about how to discover the unique values of the client, how to identify self-defeating influences in their lives, and how to create a vision for the future.
- Balance: Trainees learn how to assist their clients in generating perspectives and in creating a plan of action grounded in commitment. In addition they are taught how to guide clients in making powerful new choices in their lives.
- Process: They also learn how to help clients with understanding life's chaos and inertia and the confusion that follows. Being with the client during this time period is said to help the clients feel known and helps them to know themselves.
- In the Bones: Intuition is encouraged in helping clients with their problems. This section of the training is said to be for the purpose of integrating the coaching skills that were learned in previous courses and to take coaching to a higher level of impact and professionalism (Certified Professional Co-Active Coach Training Institute, 2012, pp. 1-2).

According to one school of coaching:

> The Bureau of Labor Statistics (BLS) classifies life coaches as social and human service assistants and finds that this occupation can anticipate a 23% job growth rate through 2018. Much of that growth will happen in private agencies and will result from factors such as greater numbers of retirees and the public's increased emphasis on personal and mental health (Natural Healers, 2012).

On this website are over 130 pages of schools and programs advertised to provide training in the United States and Canada. Some are for coaching, some for chiropractic medicine, alternative medicine, the healing arts, and massage therapy. Schools are listed by state including schools in Costa Rica. Another program offers certifications in the following:

- Professional
- Life
- Business
- Career
- Executive
- Bereavement
- Addiction
- Wellness
- Spiritual
- Christian
- Marketing
- Mentor

- Master
- Youth
- Family
- Parent

At best there are a number of programs attached to universities and at worst many cottage industry types of programs fishing for customers. The top programs will assist the trainee in setting up their website and Pay Pal program along with ways to create ads and where to place them on the Internet. For the licensed professional, this might be an opportunity worth exploring. It can be a part-time position that might build into a more lucrative business. There are few of the risks and liabilities of health care practice, and there are fewer changes, fewer no-shows and it is a home-based business with no additional overhead expenses. You can use your computer and Internet systems and a bank account for Pay Pal deposits. If one can talk to someone in the business, the inside information might lower some of the concerns and save some costly experiments.

SERVITUDE

Servitude can be defined as an individual who feels subjected, voluntarily or involuntarily, to another person, corporation, HMO, or state, as a servant or one who has no value only as defined by the corporation or state. While there are important similarities with those who work as servants for others, most providers would like to believe that they are independent and free of the chains of servitude. Health care providers are waking up to a new relationship with the state and federal governments and their appointed managers, HMOs. We do have a choice. However, it may mean breaking free of managed care and the state run reimbursement program and only accepting cash.

A growing number of psychologists, psychiatrists, PCPs, and therapists are trying a new model of delivery. Physicians are just as frustrated as other providers. By accepting only cash payments they can lower their costs and the number of patients they have to see each day, thus giving them more personal time with their families and hobbies. It also removes the gorilla on their back that is felt when having to accept Big Brother in the room as well as the risks of recoupment and disruptions of new practice rules sent down from state and federal government agencies. The physicians and psychologists feel more in control again and the nightmares have evaporated. Providers that are cash based have different ways they operate, such as charging a monthly retainer fee plus $10 for each visit or $100 for a more involved service. Some will guarantee that they will respond within 12 to 24 hours, others promise to return a call at night if needed. For those without insurance this can be a great option. For those with insurance but who are unhappy with treatment by their HMO provider, this can be a welcome alternative.

When the federal and state governments unite against health care providers they are also controlling the futures of patients and the practitioners. The basic assumption of this management by leverage (or Theory L) are the needs of the MCOs and HMOs take precedence over the rights of physicians, hospitals, nurses, social workers, psychologists, psychotherapists, physical therapists, occupational therapists, respiratory therapists, and other allied care providers including the pharmaceutical corporations. In other words, the people deliver the goods, in addition to the patients who are, for the most part, taxpayers who are obligated to pay for whatever the government tells them to pay. Remember how President Bush was able to create a *second army* in the Middle East? He did it by paying contractors to do chores that would free up the military to focus on the actual battlefield exchanges. The costs for these contractors have reached new heights of spending that are now bloating the national debt. Within the battle for control of the health care industry the Department of Health and Human Services is creating a whole new extension of government through their division of government as well as the judicial and law enforcement agencies with the Justice Department and the Homeland Security Department. The contractors are the HMOs, the recruitment administrators for the HMOs, and the security or fraud division of the HMOs.

Today the reform movement takes away the rights of professional providers to define and control their practices. The Act of 2010 promises to add even more controls, including putting case managers in physician offices. Cutting reimbursement rates is a way to drive out providers who would be rebels and could be uncooperative. Withholding adequate and timely information to practices and hospitals is a weapon in HMOs and state governments that will drive providers away because they need timely information to survive change. Sending auditors or investigating providers and not giving adequate and timely information as to why there is an investigation or audit, and what their rights are prior to the start of the audit or investigation will drive providers out, too. These are only a few ways that can demoralize the present providers of health care services. There have been shortages of medical, nursing, and mental health providers for over 40 years and now they are attempting to force them to move on so that there will be less accessibility of services to a majority of those living in rural or border communities all across the nation. It will be easier for a Native American to obtain quality health care than an American born in West Texas who is disabled.

A right is an entitlement. If I have a right to medical care, then I am entitled to the time, the effort, the ability, the wealth, of whoever is going to be forced to provide that care. In other words, I own a piece of the taxpayers who subsidize me. I own a piece of the doctors who tend to me. The notion of a right to medical care goes far beyond any notion of charity. A doctor who waives his bill because I am indigent is offering a free gift; he retains his autonomy, and I owe him gratitude. But if I have a right to care, then he is merely giving me my due, and I owe him nothing. If others are forced to serve me in the name of my right to care, then they are being used regardless of their will as a means to my welfare. I am stressing this point because many people do not appreciate that the very concept of welfare rights, including the right to health care, is incompatible with the view of individuals as ends in themselves (Kelly, 2012, p. 4-5).

Kelley quotes Ayn Rand from her novel, *The Fountainhead*: "Men have been taught that the highest virtue is not to achieve, but to give. Yet one cannot give that which has not been created. Creation comes before distribution—or there will be nothing to distribute. The need of the creator comes before the need of any possible beneficiary" (Kelley, 2012 p.9). According to Dr. Kelly the needs of a creator of goods or services, is to exercise their freedom to act as they were trained (it was their money that paid for their education), the freedom to share or sell their knowledge the way they choose, and the freedom to interact with others on a voluntary basis, by trade and mutual exchange which is currently illegal. Currently providers cannot even barter with a patient without jeopardizing their license.

In 1993 Dr. Kelly spoke to these issues and they are more relevant today than they were 20 years ago. To summarize, a political system that tries to implement a right to health care will necessarily involve: forced transfers of wealth to pay for programs, loss of freedom for health care providers, higher prices and more restricted access for all consumers, a trend toward egalitarianism, and the collectivization of health care. These consequences are not accidental as they are derived from the basic nature of the alleged *right*.

CONCLUSION

Control is an underlying force that pushes and is pushed back as states fight with the federal government, providers push back against the weight of threats to their practices, and patients push back against being bumped from one Medicaid plan to an HMO plan. The HMOs have invested billions in winning a large population to administer insurance claims and policies and they have hired layers of case managers and other filter builders to delay payments, to cut entitlements, and to encourage providers to fall into line behind their leadership. The stakes are high and they see the writing on the wall. The new configuration of MCOs to HMOs is a step toward single payer policies within the next decade.

Managed care, as a business, is supported by the state and federal law enforcement communities. If a loan is defaulted, the bank cannot, at least at this time, send their name to a law enforcement organization and have the family evicted or harassed at the point of a gun and the presence of a badge. Eviction notices and eviction processes are administered by sheriff deputies in many cases. Large grocery chains do not have the ability to call authorities if food goes bad quicker than expected, it is simply a cost of doing business. Department stores exercise the right to protect themselves against losses, such as pilferage, with a security group. Educational institutions now have their own police departments; some housing communities hire a security force to guard their homes and property.

Over the next 10 years there will be an increase in shortages of primary care physicians and mental health providers, and an increase in providers from other countries being given work permits and visas and qualifying to fill these shortages. Secondly, some graduate schools may look for alternative course work that addresses these issues and that supports legislative changes in licensing requirements. By 2024 it is reasonable to expect that every health care provider, outside of hospital corporations, will be working in a civil servant position unless they work outside of any license. One of the first steps to independence is to stop taking insurance coverage and secondly, consider turning your license back to the state. There is a growing number of practices only accepting cash. Physicians are offering a monthly payment plan where people who can afford to pay from $25 to $75 a month can be assured that the physician will call them within a certain amount of time. Secondly, the physician rates will be within a range they can afford and the physician sometimes offers to accept monthly payments on top of the regular monthly fee for having this relationship. Coaching, mentoring, and consultations may be the future for those feeling pinched out of a position at the table of funding.

As political entities change at state and federal levels there is always an opportunity for a change in direction and in priorities of the national voice. Which means that an option not discussed in this chapter may come to the surface at any time when there is a political groundswell for change again. One would be foolish not to include such an option when considering changing one's career path. In the end, the search for satisfaction, for internal balance, is a never-ending quest for those passionate about life.

Chapter Six

The Future of Healthcare

The purpose of this chapter is to examine the current obdurate movements of healthcare reform through the eyes of those perplexed about all the changes of the current system who are asking, "what's next?" This chapter analyzes several factors that address the value of futurism projections. This approach is natural to researchers as a way to anticipate future needs of society that decision makers of every discipline can use and apply to their institution, corporation, or governmental agency. For public health care researchers it is second nature to plan ahead because the basic core of public health service is prevention, something that separates them from the physical medicine approach.

In the first chapter we addressed the effects of the healthcare reform on providers. In chapter two we exposed the notion that private practice was private and providers have little or no autonomy, as was experienced in the previous century. The third chapter focused on the obstacles for providers within the practice of healthcare. In the fourth chapter we tackled the multiple hats that practitioners are wearing at any given time. In the fifth chapter we suggest some ways to increase the value of service as a way to increase personal energy that can restore the passion for quality. As we acknowledge the third anniversary of the ACT, we must watch as the dust falls from the impact of the other shoe falling (Brill's pill), and question the morality of our choices, the ephemerality of our dreams.

According to the Department of Health and Human Services:

- About 71 million Americans in private health insurance plans received coverage in 2011 and 2012 for at least one free preventive health care service, such as a mammogram or flu shot.

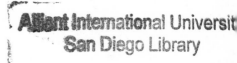

- Another estimated 34 million Medicare beneficiaries have paid nothing out of pocket for at least one preventive service, such as an annual wellness visit.
- More than 3.1 million young adults are now covered with some type of insurance, since they can stay on their parents' policies until age 26.
- Approximately 105 million Americans no longer face lifetime limits on their coverage. Starting in 2014 annual limits will also be prohibited.
- The Prevention and Public Health Fund provided $2.25 billion for state and local public health activities in fiscal years 2010-2012, and $1 billion is available through the fund in fiscal year 2013, though sequestration will reduce the fund by $51 million over the remainder of the year.
- 8,500 community health centers have received funding to provide care to their communities (Department of Health and Human Services, 2013).

While these are *feel goods*, they did not reduce health care costs, did not increase access goals, and did nothing to increase quality of services and to decrease disparities. The problem of inadequate or no insurance is just as bad now as it was in 2009. People that have no insurance are waiting as long as possible and then will go to the nearest ER or doctor's office asking for help. An example of this was Luis, 51, who worked for a company in Texas for years, and his employer terminated his insurance. One day Luis drove 200 miles for a consultation with a specialist in Houston. The doctor who performed the free screening then told him that he needed an operation, as his colon cancer had advanced.

"Seventy percent of the people we see here are employed," said Dr. G. Bobby Kapur, associate chief of the emergency room at Ben Taub General Hospital, part of the taxpayer-supported Harris Hospital District. "They're hourly wage earners, nannies, people working in lawn care services or dry cleaners or real estate, or people working two part-time jobs and neither will pay the health care," he said. "Many are small business owners who are well educated and well dressed" (Rabin, 2012, p. 1).

The ACT, which is said to provide over 32 million people with health care insurance over the next five years, will start in 2014 and extend to 2019, and even then there will still be some left on the outside looking in. (Silberman, Liao, Ricketts, 2010, p. 215). Many will receive eligibility through Medicaid, others through extensions for insurance that can be purchased at a reduced rate based on the family income; however, not every American will be covered. The ACT expands coverage to most Americans through low-income programs by encouraging employers to purchase group coverage or to extend or increase coverage through financial incentives. The ACT also creates a scenario where small businesses can purchase affordable coverage through directly given financial incentives (p. 216). The ACT does this through collaborations with states on extensions, but also through direct appropriations and authorizations. Appropriation means the funding is available immediately, while authorizations are programs that will receive funding in the future. The remaining people not covered, or who cannot afford health care premiums through extensions, may have to wait longer for accessibility to quality health care. This raises the question of the *right* to healthcare.

Politics does have an impact on social policies. Politicians are sensitive to criticism in the media as they are afraid of their deep pocket supporters who might decide to back another candidate next election. Ideas are what shape positions those politicians and bureaucrats (who write the legislative bills and can put their biases within the law) lust for which "shapes political alliances and strategic considerations of building and maintaining alliances. Ideas and portrayals are key forms of power in power making" (Stone, 2002, p. 34). Healthcare providers tend to shy away from politics as they see it as something beneath their dignity; however, politics is very active in the healthcare policy decisions and reform changes. Just like providers who never really appreciated the business side of medicine or therapy, there is now the politics of medicine and therapy that is pushing providers around by forcing them to change their practices and putting more auditors and case managers in the offices of providers.

Sheldon (2011) is a professor and researcher in the Department of Surgery and Social Medicine at the University of North Carolina at Chapel Hill. He advocates for the goal of a high-quality healthcare system, but also acknowledges that this will require immediate attention to physicians, surgeons, nurses, and other health care providers now in short supply. It should be understood that health care costs are likely to increase. The alternative is rationing. The challenge is to find revenue sources and payment methods and to maximize the efficiency and equity of the system (p. 1110).

With constant changes from a variety of sources within the three domains of public health services there is bound to be frustration, confusion, and shortages. Sheldon is an advocate for health care for everyone, calling it "a right and a positive good. Quality of health care supports the stability and quality of a society" (p. 1104). Reaching the goals of quality control and accessibility for all will take some time working through the financial and administrative issues, and, in the meantime, patients, providers, insurers, government agencies, and state bureaucracies will have to continue with the tug-of-war between issues of debates of individualism and socialism labels.

The ACT was also created to decrease disparities in access and in quality of service. Brody, Glenn, and Hermer have reviewed health care disparities since the ACT was legislated and they suggest a multi-level approach to correcting the problem of disparities. Their argument is that racial and ethnic questions are often "dismissed from the larger discussions of socioeconomic inequities" (2012, p. 309), as if there is "no useful role for a bioethicist at the table" to discuss policy development (p. 309). An example is in clarification of the definitions of "race" and "ethnic" where there is often confusion. "Even skilled genomics investigators, for instance, may be indefensibly sloppy in describing their methods, if any, for deciding who is of what race or ethnicity" (p.309). In the collection of surveys or information from charts the term "race" may not "fit" everyone the same because of major genetic or biological differences. The classic "race" that has been divided into a few "types" has long been disproven as a legitimate biological category and has been thoroughly discredited as a tool of medical research (p.309). This has implications for surveillance and survey research investigations as well as established data collections at community, state, and federal levels. For example, how can the color of skin be considered a race, and yet a person who is white is given the choice of "white" or "caucasian." No article has been written, that this author has seen, which explains from what country produces caucasians.

Snowden, McGeary, Kunerth, Carlson, McRae, and Vetta (2012) offer a way to address disparities with an instrument that has been successful in Minnesota. This instrument is the Minnesota Health Care Disparities Report, which was designed to meet the reporting needs of the insurers. The authors suggest that this tool meets the needs of confidentiality and accurate reporting of data that improves transparency in the delivery of healthcare. The authors present a tool that has had success in identifying and reporting disparities in the delivery of health services. Those considered being from a low social economic status (SES) often have no access to prenatal services. Other disparities include the lack of immunization and preventive care, fewer papanicolaou tests, mammograms, lack of services for asthma and depression, and diabetic eye examinations (p. 275). In addition children of lower SES families often have more problems with behavior, take more risks, and can have earlier contact with law enforcement than those not of lower SES families.

Shortages have been growing within a number of professional specialties within the healthcare delivery system. The Hogg Foundation (2011) at the University of Texas in Austin has been in operation since 1940 and has specialized in adding to the awareness of the public and academia of the value of health care services and the mental health needs within the state of Texas. They document the shortage in Texas of mental health providers, mapping out the shortages by counties. There are many counties without a psychiatrist, psychologist, licensed professional counselor, or a licensed marriage and family therapist. They serve as a prodder of political conscious by being in the bottom level of states that provide funding for mental health disorders. Given the changes brought on by the ACT, insurers are working with states to eliminate fee-for-service providers, in other words, those in private practice. Half of those in private practice in Texas have left the profession in the past 18 months and others are finding work in government as well as in community mental health or non-profit organizations.

Primary care physicians are feeling the squeeze applied to them by HMOs and state Medicaid systems that are pushing fee-for-services health care practices into group practices, or Affordable Care Organizations, also known as medical homes, and Coordinated Care Organizations which are a network of providers clinging onto their individual practices, but working as a loosely formed group to provide the quality of care and utilization review that HMOs and the ACT require. A physician addressed what he views as happening to American physicians:

> These changes in medical knowledge, healthcare delivery, and technology have brought about the creative destruction of American family practice and times and circumstances dictate it will go the way of performing an appendectomy on the kitchen table, house calls, and the hometown doctor of a Norman Rockwell illustration (Brooks, 2013).

Pharmacies are another group that has been hit hard by the new regulations that seem to be driving many out of business. Thompson (2011) reports on why pharmaceutical medications are being reimbursed to some pharmacies. With an influx of patients that will be covered by some health care insurance over the next 18 months there is concern in the pharmaceutical industry that they may not be prepared to meet the expected demand due to the fact that small family pharmacies are being driven out of business by mega corporations with contracts from insurers that family pharmacies lack. Other shortages are occurring in dentistry, chiropractic medicine, and home health care. While these are important, space does not allow for more in depth discussion and documentation of each profession that is facing significant shortages. Shortages in any profession decrease accessibility and are detrimental to the goals of ACT.

Three nurses have written about their concern for what they anticipate as a shortage of nurses by 2020. They argue that many of the current nurses have Registered Nurse (RN) licenses but only have an associate's degree. In today's market nurses are required to have at least a Bachelor's degree with a RN license (Reilly, Fargen, and Walker-Daniels, 2011). "In light of a predicted general shortage of one million nurses by 2020, the Institute of Medicine, in its recent Future of Nursing report, stressed the importance of attracting and retaining well-prepared nurses in multiple care settings, including those in public health. Although a bachelor of science in nursing degree (BSN) isn't universally required for entry into public health nursing, it's practically essential (p. 11). Koh and Jacobson (2009) address the need for positive and active leadership among the public health practitioners. Koh is the Harvey V. Fineberg Professor of the Practice of Public Health and an

Associate Dean for Public Health Practice while Jacobson is the Executive Director of Leadership Initiatives at the Division of Public Health Practice, Harvard School of Public Health, Boston, MA. Reinhard and Hassmiller are researchers with the American Association of Retired People (AARP) where they research and write on public policy, including championing the cause of the nursing profession in America. They address this shortage and the possible impact on access to health care. In addition, they suggest that hospitals of the future will have their fees substantially reduced as the costs of health care rise substantially within a medical/hospital institution vs. a primary care clinic or office.

Prior to the ACT the problems that were pounded by the media and the legislative leaders included access, quality of care, and costs. Access refers to those that were underinsured or not insured due to social economic status (SES) and are possibly living in rural and border communities where transportation to a larger city challenged their pocketbooks and the distant travel discouraged more than one trip. Access also includes disparities within health care and the lack of parity between medical and mental health services provided by insurers despite the legislation of parity six years ago. Quality of care often refers to rural and border communities where there is a shortage of specialties including nurses and mental health practitioners. These issues continue three years after the ACT was legislated and the promised land is nowhere on the horizon.

WILL THE FUTURE CHANGE THESE TRENDS?

Some have predicted a national healthcare system where everyone is covered and there is only one payer. While some argue that Medicare is better prepared than any HMO or Medicaid program to handle the sole payer role, it is only a guess as to how effective Medicare will be once in that role. Shortages of providers are encouraging Congress to accept more foreign trained physicians such as from India. In recent years it has been interesting to watch as the powers in charge have been accepting more physicians from India and Pakistan than from any Latino country. Society and Congress need to be more vigilant in protecting cultural and language issues within the practice of healthcare.

Payment reimbursement issues are not going away. The National Commission on Physician Payment Reform issued a report in March 2013 that discussed a five year plan to move from fee-for-service to a flat fee reimbursement rate or a salary position. There is no National Commission of Psychologists or master level therapists and therefore, it can only be guessed that if the physicians are going to become salaried, so is everyone else. This means that a salary will not be sufficient to support an independent practice

(IPA/CCO). ACOs and hospital providers will be the few lucky ones unless more changes are announced during the next six years.

There are many signals that sound an alarm of trends expected over the next eleven or twelve years. One alarm is the change in the way patients view their health care needs. A discussion of future health care reform movements is not necessarily a discussion of the needs of the people, since decision makers frequently group people into a clan of weepers and complainers (Keegan, 2013), physicians as wanting more money, and corporate leaders demanding lower health insurance premiums. A survey was taken two years ago and patients were asked what they wanted in a health care reform package (Shaywitz, 2011). A majority reported that the top five things they wanted were: to be well when sick, timeliness, kindness, hope, certainty, and continuity of care from the same doctor or team. The five things that they had little or no concern with were: percent of GNP devoted to healthcare, costs they do not bear, conflicts of interest for their providers, and equity (they were not concerned with everyone else being able to have the same type of services they had).

Another signal is the security blanket of knowing your doctor and having access to your doctor during your crisis. What we have now is the primary care physician who sees patients as needed, or as a follow-up. While some reports like the Cochrane Mega Analysis, suggested the office visit is the least efficient service; some would argue that it is the most cost effective service provided today. People need a person to talk to, to ask them the right questions that are needed to rule out various illnesses, or to monitor progress of medication or treatment. Dr. Campbell argues that:

> Outcomes are improved when patients are actively engaged in their own healthcare. Part of engagement involves forming a relationship with a physician through regular follow up visits. Relationships with doctors, just as with friends and spouses, evolve over time. Trust and communication skills are built through recurrent contact and interaction (Hill, 2013; The Cochran Collaboration, 2013, p. 1).

Primary care physicians do their best to help their patients understand risk and procedures in determining whether to have a surgical procedure, to start a new medication, or to choose not to have anything done at the present time. The literature often discusses the need to share with the physician completely and truthfully regarding aches, pains, compliance, and fears. The Cochrane Group has been testing this theory for reliability and validity.

> From three trials specifically measuring 'informed choice' as an outcome, the researchers found that when risk profiles were included in the intervention, the participants made more informed decisions about screening, compared to people who were provided with more general risk information. Overall 45.2%

(592/1309) of participants who received personalized risk information made informed choices, as compared to 20.2% (229/1135) of participants who received generic risk information. An 'informed decision' was considered as one that was consistent between knowledge, attitude and choice (Cochran, 2013, p. 1).

When futurists study the global trends, they begin with the past, going back 10 to 20 years, not only to analyze the waves of change within the profession, but also the global changes such as climate changes, immigration patterns, the graduation numbers for medical doctors and nurses in other countries that can be recruited to meet the shortages in the United States. The following study demonstrates how researchers use past trends to project future patterns.

> Ten years ago we identified a fundamental shift in the composition of the registered nurse (RN) workforce. Unless this trend was reversed, the size of the RN workforce was projected to eventually decrease as large numbers of registered nurses would retire and not be replaced by younger cohorts. Using estimates that were available at the time of the future need for registered nurses, shortfalls of 20%, or approximately 400,000 RNs, were expected by 2020. These shortfalls grew even larger when those requirements were subsequently updated (Auerbach, Buerhaus, Stalger, 2011, p. 2287).

For states that accepted the Medicaid expansion, preparation has begun. The process of identification and assessment of eligibility will begin in the last three months of 2013. For those states that did not accept the expansion, such as Texas, those without health care coverage will continue that way until there is a legislative change or until every ER becomes too crowded to breathe.

> Other health care reform changes are already underway in the public and private sectors. Testing of new methods for organizing and funding care in the areas of chronic medical conditions and potentially avoidable complications provides a window into how general healthcare reform will occur. Medical homes are being piloted to manage the health status of persons with chronic medical conditions, while bundled payment pilots are testing risk and reward arrangements for acute care episodes. Together, these types of efforts are leading to three fundamental system improvements—healthcare will become better coordinated; prevention, early intervention, and disease management services will grow with a corresponding decline in secondary and tertiary care; and errors and overuse will be disincentivized (sic) by replacing fee for service payments with risk and reward financial arrangements (National Council for Community Behavioral Healthcare, 2013, p, 3).

As independent professional associations (IPA) are created, members are finding that they have to pay for the expenses to run an IPA and that hiring an experienced attorney to seam-up an attractive package has utility for both producers and patients, but it takes money. Each organization is then present-ed to the state organization that authorizes them to act as an IPA group of independent providers within the guidelines of the state. There is lots of paperwork to be done and the group must work together, not only to pay the bills, but to understand the process. Recently one group found that their state was defining *therapy* per the DSM-V. Many therapists who understand the nature of group experiences and background have argued that there are built-in biases favoring therapy by medicine over psychotherapy, and that has created many concerns. In other words, along the way to accreditation there are bumps in the road, and there will be more.

Another bump in the road are the audits that each HMO is preparing to initiate. One HMO group shared their list of questions for an audit of mental health providers and the list had over 85 questions. When a provider receives a list of names and dates to send to the recoupment department or the man-aged care department, do not be fooled. Every piece of paper in the chart should be included as every progress note, or referral letter, or assessment is part of the total package that addresses documentation and compliance is-sues. Too many providers have only sent the requested dates and progress notes and have received requests for a check to reimburse the HMO because of a lack of adequate documentation. Each group or individual provider has the right to ask for a copy from each HMO they are paneled. If an organiza-tion fails to respond or refuses to send the provider or group a copy, put their name on the professional list service, and second, contact your group's legal representation for advice. Providers have a right to this information, but HMOs have never been good at recognizing the value of collaborating with providers in order to ensure quality. Their frame of mind is to "catch" provid-ers in a mistake and to turn their name in to the organization's legal depart-ment for an audit or legal action. Belonging to a professional list service helps spread the news about these companies who are trying to run over the providers in order to save money. The more they save, the bigger their bonuses are with the state!

Public health is all about prevention; therefore, being prepared means being in a position to understand the possible effects of any health threat or environmental change that can have an impact on air, land, water, food, and health. There are the normal changes of life, such as the aging populations who will require more services in their senior years even though they have been relatively healthy all their lives. Secondly, there are the growing issues, beginning in childhood, of obesity and chronic diseases such as diabetes. Thirdly, there are still issues of inequitable health care systems and the threat of infectious diseases that can spread rapidly. According to Curbow and Hanson (2010) we can anticipate, but cannot predict, the timing or the region with much accuracy, such as water shortages, climate changes, new technology, wars, hurricanes and tornados, or economic fluctuations that can stab the heart of investors and corporation leaders with fear and anxiety.

While the investor and corporate leaders fret and worry about upturns and downturns of the market, the common man and woman are worried about their next paycheck. Therefore, when corporations on Wall Street charge President Obama with attempts to change our democratic system of government to socialism, the common man and woman may have a different perspective and are not as likely to worry about the terms.

A recent Pew Research Center poll found that a majority of Americans have an unfavorable view of corporations—a significant shift from only twelve years ago, when nearly three-quarters held a favorable view. At the same time, two recent Rasmussen surveys found Americans under the age of 30—the people who will help build the next political arena—almost equally divided as to whether capitalism or socialism is preferable. Another Pew survey found that 18 to 29-year-olds have a favorable reaction to the term "socialism" by a margin of 49 to 43 percent (Alpreovitz and Hanna, 2012).

The talk of public ownership of the health care industry is seen as a better option with funding corporations being gatekeepers on health care matters when the corporation's number one obligation to their shareholders is to make a profit. The government operates from a different perspective, which can bring these issues into the public debate. Alperovitz and Hanna document how corporations have always resisted comprehensive curbs on environmental hazards such as gas emissions (p. 18) and have taken advantage of tax loopholes to keep from paying taxes and pushing the limits of anti-trust regulations (p.19). Alperovitz is the Lionel R. Bauman Professor of Political Economy at the University of Maryland and co-founder of the Democracy Collaborative and the author of *America Beyond Capitalism*. Hanna is the senior research assistant at the Democracy Collaborative. Their work underlines their concern that the takeover of the health care industry by corporations can only lead to more centrality of corporate power, at least during this present time, hurting health care by destroying private practice and increasing the disparities of access and quality.

THE OTHER SHOE

A lot of time has been taken, millions of words written, about the need for Americans to take responsibility for their own lifestyles to decrease healthcare costs by creating ways to eat healthier, exercise more, and reduce toxins to the system and to lifestyles (alcohol, drugs, and risky behaviors). The ACT was created, in part, to force providers of all healthcare services to change from their present way of billing and delivery, to one that was considered the best type of delivery of service (group practices). All those in private practice are in a fee-for-service billing format. The insurers limit what is allowed from their policies. In a growing number of states where Medicaid has sold out administrative services to HMOs the reimbursement rate decreases to Medicaid rates and, as state legislators endorse decreasing rates, the providers have to accept the lower rates or stop seeing patients with Medicaid rates. For those in rural communities, where 95% of the population may be on Medicaid, this creates a scenario where providers have to close their practice. With more and more shortages, patients with Medicaid policies are traveling two hours or more to find a provider who will accept their coverage. With metropolitan community providers seeing more of these long distance travelers, there are two warnings: if the patient doesn't keep their appointment, they may not receive a referral or a follow-up appointment; secondly, patients are placed on waiting lists that can extend for six months or longer. The bottom line is that access to health care providers is decreasing rather than increasing as promised by the ACT. The ones hit the hardest are those in rural and border communities.

Those in private practice of health care, home health care, dentistry, chiropractic medicine, and some primary care physicians have been closing their offices over the past 18 months. They have had to close their practices because state Medicaid and HMO reimbursement rates have fallen steadily, plus there has been an increase in recoupment activity and audits that interfere with practice and cut-off funds needed in order to keep the lights on. Over the last three years the focus of state law enforcement integrity teams has been to force fee-for-service practices to close, while the real culprits in the rising costs equation are public and non-profit HOSPITALS. Until now.

In a special report by *Time* magazine, March 4, 2013, Steven Brill puts his finger on hospitals as the real vulture of patient and corporate wallets. Brill has been the first one to step up to the plate and swing at the giants of the health care industry that overcharge by trillions of dollars each year in order that they may pay their senior executives millions of dollars in bonuses each year. Even if they are a non-profit facility, this does not hamper the executives from making millions of dollars at the expense of patients who cannot defend themselves against the collection agencies of the hospitals.

> What protects the hospitals against the ACT and other attempts at cutting their rates? Lobbyists! "According to the Center for Responsible Politics, the pharmaceutical and healthcare product industries, combined with organizations representing doctors, hospitals, nursing homes, health services and HMOs, have spent $5.36 billion since 1998 on lobbying in Washington. That dwarfs the $1.53 billion spent by the defense and aerospace industries and the $1.53 billion spent by the oil and gas industries over the same period" (Brill, 2013, p. 20).

Brill reports that there are seven lobbyists, working for some segment of health care, for every member of Congress. In addition, Brill reports that the costs of services and procedures have increased over four times and now fees are over 11% profit, which is the revenue after operating expenses have been covered. Examples include blood tests: a CBC may cost Medicare $11.02 but non-Medicare patients are often charged $157.61. Medicare pays $23.83 for each X-ray, but hospitals charge $333 for each one and they can take as many X-rays as they want without being questioned. Stress tests are another example: Medicare pays $554 while hospitals charge everyone else $7,997.54 (Brill, pp.22-33). Primary care physicians are charging $125 for an office visit and they can fit in six of them per hour. However, a CBC can be done in less than five minutes and a hospital can do hundreds a day. Stress tests may take 30 minutes but in the hospital hundreds are done every day. Primary care physicians are extremely limited in what they can charge and what they can charge for; the same is true for psychotherapists who can only see 12 patients a day and while a psychologist can charge $160 an hour to a cash patient, Medicaid will pay closer to $65. This means that psychotherapists who have a master's degree are now getting $45 per hour for a Medicaid patient and they can only charge for 12 per day. Mental health providers cannot pay overhead expenses on these low rates. States say they have to cut back, Washington agrees, but they are cutting back on those who get the lowest fees! They are doing this because mental health providers lack revenues to pay for slick lobbyists and attorneys. On the other hand, hospitals, profit and not-for-profit do have these resources and have been left alone. Many are paying their CEOs, COOs, CFOs and other top executives millions of dollars in salaries and bonuses each year because their organizations, such as Sloan-Kettering, MD Anderson (pp. 24-26), and other cancer medical centers have so much money that they can build 18 floor medical clinics in downtown Dallas, Los Angeles, Atlanta, Miami, New York City, and other metropolitan communities, as well as buy advertising time on all channels in the United States and in many foreign countries.

The Brill article also clearly presented how hospitals were not the only ones inflating prices, such as charging one patient $49,237 for a Medtronic stimulator which is estimated to be over 150 percent of cost. The hospital was Mercy Hospital, which is under the umbrella of the Catholic Church called Sisters of Mercy. The patient's total expense at the hospital was over $86,950 (Brill, p. 33). According to the article the "Oklahoma City unit of the Sisters of Mercy hospital chain collected $337 million in revenue for the fiscal year ending June 30, 2012. It had an operating profit of $34 million. And that was after paying ten executives more than $300,000 each, including $784,000 to a regional president and $438,000 to the hospital president (p. 33). Brill's article is well documented and reveals lopsidedness to President Obama's Affordable Care Act of 2010. Mercy Hospital is not the sole case.

The practice of overcharging patients was created by a position in large medical centers called the Chargemaster. Leaving hospitals out of the mix is like the debate that President Obama had with Mitt Romney about asking everyone to share in the loss of some benefits including increasing the taxes of the super rich. Apparently President Obama and CMS have forgotten the elites of healthcare billing when it comes to cutting healthcare costs. It is hard to believe that nothing has been done up to this point. It is not that CMS does not want to tackle this issue, but they feel that Congress is holding them back because Congress is feeling the pressure of special interests supporting mega health centers.

What might happen now? This question has a multitude of available responses; none of them may be exactly the way things turn out in three, seven, or even fifteen years. Bloggers and researchers alike have an opinion based on their experiences, a conversation with a CMS employee or another "deep throat." I have read articles suggesting that Blue Cross and Blue Shield will take over the sole provider role when the time comes. I have also heard that the federal government will be the payer, perhaps using Medicare, but might also farm out regional contracts, if not to bureaucrats, then to HMO managers and utility control personnel to handle regions within each state for administration and insurance fraud tasks. One might hope that CMS forces the debate into the legislative halls and into the nightly newscasts and on the Sunday morning talk shows. The idea being that more input and discussions need to be generated within the middle class and others rather than with just lobbyists or blue ribbon committees as they have virtually little awareness of what others are thinking about or needing. Elitism is normally narrowly funneled and narcissistic, as those who are social advocates might also be viewed. Secondly, the government has a civil service structure that may be able to absorb health care providers. Thirdly, the American Public Healthcare System comes out of the Department of Health and Human Services and has a structure and a history of prevention and research that reaches from the local communities, to state and federal government, as well as global governments. The public healthcare service is capable of providing the regional staffs and locations to handle many of the administrative and billing issues of a local service, in addition to understanding the cultural, financial, and language barriers that often impede the implementation of quality within healthcare prevention, education, and treatment. Taking all the money paid to law enforcement officials in each HMO, MCO, and state government could be used to streamline the system and reduce administrative costs. Medicare administration of health care is about $3 per case where other organizations are charging over ten times that amount.

At the beginning of this book the question was postured: Why isn't healthcare based on fundamental moral principles as much as on questions of healthcare quality? Now, at the end, we must ask, are we any closer to reaching a gratifying solution? Working towards this goal is like working for the improvement of a safer and healthier society. However, it will take a significant reduction of the bully approach to management of providers to begin that process. The theory of leverage may work in corporate board rooms but providers have a different mentality and that is not all bad. Providers are not the enemy; they are the body and soul of quality caring health treatments. If HMOs and state bureaucrats could find a way to work together with providers, to include a two-way stream of communication, there may be fewer shortages, goals of quality care may return in practice, and patients may find access returning again. The health care industry needs to return to its roots in order to regain their dignity and the trust of the populations they serve.

References

AAPC. (2012). CMS starts immediate recoupment for overpayments. http://news.aapc.com/index.php/2012/02/cms-starts-immediate-recoupment-for-overpayments/.

Ackley, D. C. (1997). *Breaking free of managed care, a step-by-step guide to regaining control of your practice.* NY: The Guilford Press.

Advertisement. (2012). *Medicaid state changes.* The News Gram, Eagle Pass, TX, April 15.

Affordable Care Act of 2010 (2012). *Goals for the next three years.* http://medicaid.gov/AffordableCareAct/Timeline/Timeline.html.

Allen, J. (2010). *Majority of Americans distrust the government.* Pew Research Center. Reuters. http://www.reuters.com/article/2010/04/19/us-americans-government-poll-dUSTRE63I0FB20100419.

Alperovitz, G., and Hanna, T. M. (2012). *Not so wild a dream.* The Nation, June 11, 18-23.

Auerbach, D. I., Buerhaus, P. I., and Staiger, D. O. (2011). *At the intersection of health, health care, and policy.* Health Affairs, *30* (12): 2286-2292. doi: 10.1377/hlthaff.2011.0588

Bernhard, Y. A. (1975). *Self-care is the process by and through which self-respect, self-worth, and self-liking are developed.* Millbrae, CA: Celestial Arts.

Barlett, D. L. and Steele, J. B. (2006). *Critical condition, how health care in America became big business – and bad medicine.* NY: Broadway Books.

Beelman, M. (2003). *U.S. contractors reap the windfalls of post-war reconstruction.* Center for Public Integrity. http://www.commondreams.org/headlines03/1030-10.htm.

Berenson, R. A. & Burton, R. A. (2011). *Accountable care organizations in Medicare and the private sector: A status update.* Robert Wood Johnson Foundation and the Urban Institute. www.rwjf.org/files/research/73470.5470.aco.report.pdf.

Bloche, M. G. (2003) (Ed). *The privatization of health care reform, Legal and regulatory perspectives.* NY: Oxford University Press.

Bodenheimer, T. (2005). *The political divide in health care: A liberal perspective.* Health Affairs, November/December 2005.

Borosage, R. L., Gerson, R. & Lotke, E. (2006 September). *War profiteers profit over patriotism in Iraq.* Retrieved December 23, 2012 from http://home.ourfuture.org/reports/report-war-profiteers.pdf.

Brill, S. (2013). *Bitter pill, how outrageous pricing and egregious profits are destroying our health care.* NY: Time Magazine, March 4, (*181*), 8, 2013.

Brodsky, S. (2001). *Testifying in court, guidelines & maxims for the expert witness.* Washington, D.C.: American Psychological Association.

Brody, H., Glenn, J. E. and Hermer, L. (2012). *Racial/ethnic health disparities and ethics, the need for a multilevel approach.* NY: Cambridge Quarterly of Healthcare Ethics, 21. doi: 10.107/S0963180112000035.

Brooks, M. (2013). *The creative destruction of the American family physician*. Kevin, M.D. blog. Retrieved on February 14 from http://www.kevinmd.com/blog/2013/02/creative-de-struction-american -destruction-american-family-physician.html.

Brownlee, S. (2007). *Overtreated: Why too much medicine is making us sicker and poorer*. NY: Bloomsbury.

Bryant, D. T. (2011). Bryant's healthcare solutions. Retrieved on March 22, 2013 from Kevinmd at http://a.collectivemedia.net/jump/kevinmd/primarycare;cat=primarycare.

Burks, J., Grissim Jr., J. and Winner, L. (1969). *Reporting from the University of California, Berkeley, to the Rolling Stones Magazine*, June 14. http://beauty-reality.com/travel/travel/sanFran/peoplespark3.html.

Burns, J. (2012). *An interview with François de Brantes*, Managed Care, November. http://www.managedcaremag.com/archives/1211/1211.qna_debrantes.html.

Callahan, D. (2003). *What price better health? Hazards of the research imperative*. Berkeley: University of California Press.

Caspi, A. Sugden, K., Moffittj, T.E. (2003). *Influence of life stress on depression: Moderation by a polymorphism in the 5-HTT gene*. Science, 2003; 301:386-389.

Certified Professional Co-Active Coach Training Institute (2012). http://www.certifiedcareercoaches.com/coaching-certification.

Chatterjee, P. (2003). Cheney's former company profits from supporting troops. CorpWatch. http://www.corpwatch.org/article.php?id=6008.

Coalition Against Insurance Fraud (2012). Insurance fraud. http://www.insurancefraud.org/white-paper-fraud-bureaus.htm.

Collins, M. and Peel, D. (2012). *Should every patient have a unique ID number for all medical records?* Wall Street Journal, January 23. http://online.wsj.com/article/SB10001424052970204124204577154661814932978.html.

Corrigan, P. (2004). *How stigma interferes with mental health care*. American Psychologist, *59*, 7, 614–625 DOI: 10.1037/0003-066X.59.7.614.

Cunningham, P. J. (2009). *Beyond parity: Primary care physicians' perspectives on access to mental health care*. Health Affairs, May/June , *28*, 3, 635-636; doi: 10.1377.

Cummings, N. A. and Cummings, J. L. (2013). *Refocused psychotherapy, as the first line intervention in behavioral health*. NY: Routledge.

Cummings, N. A. and O'Donohue, W. T. (2008). *Eleven blunders that cripple psychotherapy in America, a remedial unblundering*. NY: Routledge.

Curbow, B. A. and Hanson, S. L. (2010). *Future of public health*. Chapter 17. Public Health Foundations: Concepts and Practices. Elena Andresen and Erin Defries Bouldin, Eds. San Francisco, CA: Jossey-Bass.

Curry, T. and Shibut, L. (2000). *The Cost of the savings and loan crisis: Truth and consequences*. FDIC Banking Review. www.fdic.gov/bank/analytical/banking/2000dec/brv13n2_2.pdf.

Cutler, D. M. (2004). *Your money or your life, strong medicine for America's health care system*. Oxford University Press.

Daschle, T., Greenberger, S., Lambrew, J. (2008). *Critical, What we can do about the health-care crisis*. NY: Thomas Dunne Books, St. Martin's Press.

Department of Health and Human Services (2013). *Outcomes of the first three years of the ACT*. American Public Health Association, March 22. http://us mg5.mail.yahoo.com/neo/launch?.rand=es87raqc16pnh.

DHHS (2011). *Reducing costs, Protecting consumers: The Affordable Care Act on the one-year anniversary of the patient's bill of rights*. http://www.healthcare.gov/law/resources/reports/patients-bill-of-rights09232011a.pdf.

DHHS (2012). *PR 1305.2. Recoupment of overpayments*. http://www.dhs.state.il.us/page.aspx?item=20787.

Dorsey, J. L. (1975). *The Health Maintenance Organization Act of 1973 (P.L. 93-222) and prepaid group practice plan*. Medical Care, *13*, 1 (January). http://en.wikipedia.org/wiki/Health_maintenance_organization.

Doyle, A. (2012). *Unemployment insurance*. About.com. http://jobsearch.about.com/od/unemployment/a/unemploymentben.htm.

Dranove, D., (2003). *What's your life worth?* NY: Prentice Hall.

Dunlap, M. (2012). *Connecting care: Coordinating care between physicians and mental health professionals.* Portland, OR. Mentor Research Institute.

Dunn and Bradstreet (2012). *Risk management and business credit.* http://www.dnb.com/risk-management/dnbi-business-credit/14909176-1.html.

Earle, R. H. and Barnes, D. J. (1999). *Independent practice for the mental health professional, Growing a private practice for the 21st century.* Philadelphia, PA: Brunner/Mazel.

Effron, L. (2012). *US mass school shooting history.* ABC News. http://abcnews.go.com/US/mass-school-shootings-history/story?id=17975571.

Elliot, V. S. (2012). *Doctors describe pressures driving them from independent practice.*

Ethics in Business (2012). *Ethics at Haliburton & KBR.* http://www.ethicsinbusiness.net/case-studies/halliburton-kbr/.

Fikac, P. (2012). *Perry wants tax break for companies permanent.* San Antonio Express-News, April 15. http://www.mysanantonio.com/news/local_news/article/Perry-wants-tax-break-for-companies-permanent-3484087.php.

Finley, D. (2012). *Druggists dreading switch in Medicaid.* San Antonio Express-News, January 26, San Antonio, TX.

Flock, E. (2011). *Time person of the year 2011: The protester.* Washington Post: blog Post. http://www.washingtonpost.com/blogs/blogpost/post/time-person-of-the-year-2011-the-protester/2011/12/14/gIQAvZtntO_blog.html.

Florida Chain, (2012). *Top secret: Florida asks to gut the medically needy program.* http://us.mc1138.mail.yahoo.com/mc/showMessage?sMid=0&filterBy=&.ran=14956855.

Fraser, J. (2010). *Mistrust of the government.* Pew Research Center. http://threatswatch.org/rapidrecon/2010/04/mistrust-of-the-government-and/.

Free Management Library (2012). *Risk management, disaster planning and protecting against crime.* http://managementhelp.org/riskmanagement/index.htm.

Friendship Development Services (200.8). *Qualified mental retardation professional – Job description.* http://www.friendshipservices.org/forms/QMRPJobDescription.pdf.

Frost, A. (2008). *The basics of psychotherapy.* Psych Central . Retrieved on March 25, 2012, http://psychcentral.com/lib/2008/the-basics-of-psychotherapy.

George, C. (2011). *Texas facing severe mental health services shortage.* http://blog.chron.com/medblog/2011/04/texas-facing-severe-mental-health-services-shortage/.

Gigantino, J. (2012). *What is comorbid?* http://www.eHow.com/info_7788760_comorbid.html#ixzz1mGVA1wV4.

Goodman, A. & Gonzalez, J. (2011). *U.S. wasting billions while tripling no-bid contracts after decade of war in Iraq, Afghanistan.* Democracy NOW! http://www.democracynow.org/2011/9/2/us_wasting_billions_while_tripling_no

Gregg, D. W. and Loomis, V. B. (1973). *Life and health insurance handbook.* 3rd Ed., Burr Ridge, IL: Richard W. Irwin, Inc., ISBN 0-256-00169-3.

Grooms, V. (2012). *South Carolina and Myrtle Beach area mental health systems preserve through stigma and shrinking budgets.* The Sun News, December 22. http://www.myrtlebeachonline.com/2012/12/22/3235742/sc-and-myrtle-beach-area-mental.html.

Hacker, S. M. (2012). *The medical entrepreneur.* http://www.themedicalentrepreneur.com

Health Affairs (2012). *Estimating fraud and abuse.* http://www.healthaffairs.org/healthpolicy-briefs/brief.php?brief_id=72.

Hogg Foundation (2012). *Crisis point*: Mental health workforce shortages in Texas. A report. http://www.hogg.utexas.edu/uploads/documents/Mental_Health_Crisis_final_032111.pdf.

Hoffer, E. (1967). *The temper of our time.* NY: Perennial Library, Harper & Row.

Holtz, J. (2011). *Everett played key part in history of prohibition.* HealdNet. http://herald-net.com/article/20110929/NEWS01/709299943.

Herzlinger, R. (2007). *Who killed health care? America's $2 trillion medical problem and the consumer-driven cure.* NY: McGraw-Hill.

Hill, S. (2013). *The knowledgeable patient: Communication and participation in health.* Quoted the results of the personalized risk communication for informed decision making about taking screening tests. http://www.cochrane.org/features/personalised-risk-communication-informed-decision-making-about-taking-screening-tests.

Hixon, T. (2012). *What entrepreneurs can do about the health care crisis.* http://www.forbes.com/sites/toddhixon/2011/09/21/what-entrepreneurs-can-do-about-the-health-care-crisis/.

Hixson, R. R. (2006). *Battered & bruised but not out.* Bloomington, IN: AuthorHouse.

Hixson, R. R. (2011). *What is moving us?* Annals of Psychotherapy & Integrative Health, *14*, 3. Springfield, MO: American Psychotherapy Association.

Hoge, M. A., Morris, J. A., Daniels, A. S., Stuart, G. W., Huey, Leighton Y., and Adams, Neal (2007). *The Texas Honor Killings.* An Action Plan for Behavioral Health Workforce Development.

Hoft, J. (2011). http://www.thegatewaypundit.com/2011/12/texas-santa-honor-killing-dallas-killer-didnt-want-daughter-dating-non-muslim/.

Hogg Foundation. (2011). *Crisis point: Mental health workforce shortages in Texas.* www.hogg.utexas.edu/upload/documents/mental health, retrieved January 31, 2013.

Hollister, J. (2007). *Mental health staffing shortages a real headache.* Job Journal. http://www.jobjournal.com/article_printer.asp?artid=2185.

Huffingtonpost.com. (2012). *Wisconsin temple shooting.* Huffington Post. http://www.huffingtonpost.com/2012/08/05/wisconsin-temple-shooting-sikh-oak-creek_n_1744761.html.

Human Resources Services Administration (2012). *Health care professional shortages.* http://bhpr.hrsa.gov/shortage/.

Hurley and Wallin (1998). *Adopting and adapting managed care for Medicaid beneficiaries.* Urban Institute: Research of Record. http://www.urban.org/url.cfm?ID=307473.

Internal Revenue Service (2010). *Examples of health care fraud.* http://www.irs.gov/compliance/enforcement/article/0,,id=213773,00.html.

Ingersoll, G. (2012). *The Fort Hood shooting case has become even more of a travesty.* Business Insider, 2012). http://www.businessinsider.com/the-fort-hood-shooting-case-has-become-even-more-of-a-travesty-2012-12.

Johnson, D. and Chaudhry, H. J. (2012). *Medical licensing and discipline in America: A history of the federation of state medical boards.* Secaucus, NJ: Lexington Books, division of the Rowman & Littlefield Publishing Group.

Johnson, T. (2012). *Healthcare costs and U.S. competitiveness.* Council on Foreign Relations. http://www.cfr.org/health-science-and-technology/healthcare-costs-us-competitiveness/p13325

Kabene, S. M., Orchard, C., Howard, J. M., Soriano, M. A. and Leduc, R. (2006). Human Resources for Health, International Journal of Mental Health Systems, *4*, 20. doi:10.1186/1478-4491-4-20

Karren, K. J., Hafen, B. Q., Smith, N. Lee, Frandsen, K. J. (2006). *Mind/body health, the effects of attitudes, emotions, and relationships.* SF, CA: Pearson/Benjamin Cummings.

Keegan, D. W. (2013). *Don't just blame doctors: Physician payment reform report.* Report of the National Commission on Physician Payment Reform. Medscape Business of Medicine. http://www.medscape.com/viewarticle/780487_2.

Kelly, D. (2012). *Is there a right to health care?* The Atlas Society. http://www.atlassociety.org/is_health_care_a_right_obamacare

Klein, G. B. (2001). *The world's first insurance company.* http://www.irmi.com/expert/articles/2001/klein07.aspx

Koh, H. K. and Jacobson, M. (2009). *Fostering public health leadership.* Journal of Public Health, 31, 2. NY: Oxford University Press. doi 10.1093

Landreth, G. L. (2002). *Play therapy: The art of relationships.* 2nd Ed., NY: Brunner-Routledge.

Lankton, S. R. (1982). *Ericksonian approaches to hypnosis and psychotherapy, essential readings.* Jeffrey K. Zeig, ED, NY: Brunner/Mazel Publishers.

Lazarus, D. (2012). *Insurers limit consumers for getting prescribed drugs.* www.latimes.com/business/la-fi-lazarus-20120504,O,4471449.

Lewis, J. M. and Hensley, T. R. (1998). *The May, 1970 shootings at Kent State University: The search for historical accuracy.* Ohio Council for the Social Studies Review, *34*, 1, Summer, pp. 9-21.

Lenihan, L. P., (1999). *Physician duty to warn third parties.* Physicians' News Digest. http://www.physiciansnews.com/law/899lenihandv.html.

Lohse, G. (2011). *Provider enrollment and the patient protection and Affordable Care Act.* http://www.caqh.org/Reform/NCVHSEnrollmentTestimonywithAttachments.pdf

Lovinger, S. L. (1998). *Child psychotherapy: From initial therapeutic contact to termination.* NJ: Jason Aronson Inc.

Lowes, R. (2012). *Medicaid raise will more than double fees in 6 states.* http://www.medscape.com/viewarticle/776399?src=wnl_edit_medn_fmed&spon=34

Lowes, R. (2012). *EHR rankings suggest 'epic' shakeout.* http://www.medscape.com/viewarticle/776269?src=nldne.

Luban, R. (1994). *Keeping the fire.* Audio cassette. Lubbock, TX: Learn, Inc.

Martin, G. (2012). *Houston-based super PAC targets incumbents in both parties.* http://www.chron.com/news/houston-texas/article/Houston-based-super-PAC-targets-incumbents-in-3362678.php.

McCaughey, B. (2009). *Doctors on health care reform.* Wall Street Journal, November 6. http://online.wsj.com/article/SB10001424052748703574604574501261650483596.html?mod=WSJ_WSJ_US_HealthCareReform26_7.

McKinnon, S. (2011). *Arizona congresswoman Gabrielle Giffords wounded in shooting.* The Arizona Central.com. http://www.azcentral.com/news/articles/2011/01/09/20110109gabrielle-giffords-arizona-shooting.html.

Miller, G. J. (1993). *Formal theory and the presidency.* In Researching the Presidency, ed. George C. Edwards III, John H. Kessel, and Bert A. Rockman. Pittsburg: University of Pittsburg Press.

Montaldo, C., (2012). *Dean Corll and the Houston Mass Murders.* About.com. http://crime.about.com/od/serial/p/dean_corll.htm.

Morgenthal, S., (2006). *Duty to warn/duty to protect.* http://www.heiselandassoc.com/Mydocs/Morgenthal%20Duty%20to%20Warn.pdf. Compare with the decision making tree on communicable disease and when a provider reaches a point of decision in the duty to warm/duty to protect. http://www.mindomo.com/mindmap/communicable-diseases-confidentiality-and-the-duty-to-warn-33323e979b74635eb888497afe723b94.

Morrison, I. (1996). *The second curve, managing the velocity of change.* NY: Ballantine Books.

Moukheiber, Z. (2012). *Is this patient privacy crusader doing more harm than good?* http://www.forbes.com/sites/zinamoukheiber/2012/05/10/is-this-patient-privacy-crusader-doing-more-harm-than-good/?feed=rss_home.

National Council for Community Behavioral Healthcare (2009). *Healthcare payment reform and the behavioral health safety net: What's on the horizon for the community behavioral health system.* Retrieved on March 13, 2013 from http://www.thenationalcouncil.org/galleries/policy-file/Healthcare%20Payment%20Reform%20Full%20Report.pdf.

NASW (2012). *Social workers and duty to warn state laws.* http://www.naswdc.org/ldf/legal_issue/2008/200802.asp?back=yes.

Natural Healers (2012). http://www.naturalhealers.com/qa/lifecoaching.html.

NBC Los Angeles (2012). *Timeline: mass shooting in California.* http://www.nbclosangeles.com/news/local/Mass-School-Shootings-in-California-List-Timeline-183548511.html.

Neumeister, L. (2012). *Bernard Madoff's brother to face victims in NY court.* ABC News. http://abcnews.go.com/US/wireStory/bernard-madoff-brother-face-victims-ny-court-18022656.

New York Times (2012). *Overview.* http://topics.nytimes.com/top/reference/timestopics/people/m/bernard_l_madoff/index.html.

Nurosurgical.com (2012). *Medical history and ethics.* http://www.neurosurgical.com/medical_history_and_ethics/history/history_of_health_insurance.htm

Offshore Group (2012). *Automotive manufacturing in Mexico: A 2012 Forecast.* http://offshoregroup.com/podcast/automotive-manufacturing-in-mexico-a-2012-forecast/.

Oregon Health Authority (2012). *Coordinated care organization implementation proposal.* House Bill 3650, Health Care Transformation, January.

Orr, B. (2012). *More doctors leave practices for hospitals.* WyomingNews. com. http://www.wyomingnews.com/articles/2012/10/21/news/01top_10-21-12.txt.

Pear, R. (2011). *As health costs soar, G.O.P. and insurers differ on cause.* New York Times. http://www.nytimes.com/2011/03/05/health/policy/05cost.html?pagewanted=all&_r=0.

Peel, D. (2010). *Your medical records aren't secure.* Wall Street Journal, March 23. http://online.wsj.com/article/SB10001424052748703580904575132111888664060.html.

Peper, E., Ancoli, S. and Quinn, M. (1983). *Mind/body integration in biofeedback.* NY: Plenum Press.

Pepitone, J. (2011). *Why occupy Wall Street isn't about a list of demands.* CNN Money. http://money.cnn.com/2011/10/12/technology/occupy_wall_street_demands/index.htm.

Porter, M. E. and Teisberg, E. O. (2006). *Redefining health care, creating value-based completion on results.* Boston, MA: Harvard Business School Press.

Poynter, D. (2007). *The expert witness handbook: Tips & techniques.* Santa Barbara, CA: Para Publishing.

Pressman, R. M. (1979). *Private practice: A handbook for the independent mental health practitioner.* NY: Gardner Press, Inc., division of John Wiley & Sons, Inc.

Privacy Rights Clearinghouse (2008). *Medical privacy in electronic age.* http://www.privacyrights.org/ar/keepmedfile.htm.

Privacy Rights Clearinghouse (2011). *Privacy rights fact sheet.* http://www.privacyrights.org/fs/fs6b-SpecReports.htm.

Rabin, R. C. (2012). *Rest of the country should take a good look at the situation in Texas.* June 21. Retrieved June 22, 2012 from http//:www.kaiserhealthnews.org/Stories/2012/Jun/21/Houston-texas-uninsured.

Rago, J. (2011). *Review & outlook.* Wall Street Journal, September 2. http://online.wsj.com/article/SB10001424053111904716604576542400805234770.html#.

Reilly, J. E., Fargen, J., and Walker-Daniels, K. K. (2011). *A public health nursing shortage, encouraging nurses to go back to school can augment this workforce.* American Journal of Nursing, July, *111*.

Relman, A. S. (2007). *A second opinion: Rescuing America's health care, a plan for universal coverage serving patients over profit.* NY: The Century Foundation, Perseus Books.

Reinhard, S.C., and Hassmiller, S.B. (2011). *Partners in solutions to the nurse faculty shortage.* AARP Public Policy, Institute Center to Champion Nursing in America. J Prof Nurs. 2011 Jul-Aug;27(4):197-201. doi: 10.1016/j.profnurs.2011.04.003.

Report of the National Commission on Physician Payment Reform (2013). Retrieved on March 11, 2013 from http://physician paymentcommission.org/org.

Robinson, J. C. (1999). *The corporate practice of medicine, competition and innovation in health care.* Berkeley: University of California Press.

Rothstein, M. A. (2011). *Who will treat Medicaid and uninsured patients? Retired providers can help.* Currents in contemporary bioethics. Journal of Law & Ethics, Spring.

Rugeley, C. (2001). *Killing spree at Killeen's Luby's left 24 dead.* The Chron. http://www.chron.com/life/article/Shooting-rampage-at-Killeen-Luby-s-left-24-dead-2037092.php.

Saporta, C. (2012). *Health care is a civil right.* Bradenton Herald. http://www.bradenton.com/2012/03/23/3957251/health-care-is-a-civil-right.html#storylink=cpy.

Shaywitz, D. (2011). *What do patients really want from health care?* Forbes. http://www.forbes.com/sites/davidshaywitz/2011/12/24/what-do-patients-really-want-from-health-care/.

Satir, V. (1964). *Conjoint family therapy: A guide to theory and technique.* Science and Behavior Books.

Schaaf, M., (2012). *Oak Creek reacts to Connecticut school shooting.* Oak Creek Patch. http://oakcreek.patch.com/articles/oak-creek-reacts-to-connecticut-school-shooting.

Schubiner, H., Betzold M. (2012). *Unlearn your pain.* Mind Body Publishing, MI: Pleasant Ridge.

Scutchfield, F. D. (2009). *Principles of Public Health Practice,* 3rd Ed., Cengage Learning.

Sheldon, G. F. (2011). *The evolving surgeon shortage in the health reform era.* Journal of Gastrointestinal Surgery, *15*. The Society for Surgery of the Alimentary Tract. NY: Springer Publishing Company. doi: 10.1007/s11605-011-1430-0.

Shin-Yi, W. and Green, A. (2000). *Projection of chronic illnesses prevalence and cost inflation*. Rand Corporation, October.

Smith, M., Segal, J., and Segal, R. (2012). *The difference between stress and burnout*. www.helpguide.org

Southern Poverty Law Center (2012). *Civil Rights Martyrs*. http://www.splcenter.org/civil-rightsmemorial/civil-rights-martyrs

Snowden, A. M., Kunerth, V., Carlson, A. M., McRae, J. A., and Vetta, E. (2012). *Addressing health care disparities using public reporting*. American Journal of Medical Quality. doi: 10.1177/1062860611424078.

Starr, P. (1982). *The social transformation of American medicine, the rise of a sovereign profession and the making of a vast industry*. NY: Basic Book, Inc., Publishers.

State Resource Center, (2012). *Medicaid data and systems information*. http://medicaid.gov/State-Resource-Center/State-Resource-Center.html).

Stevens, L. (2009). http://sci.tech-archive.net/Archive/sci.med/2009-06/msg00085.html

Taylor, S.E. (2010). *Mechanisms linking early life stress to adult health outcomes*. Proc Natl Acad Sci USA; 107:8507-8512.

Terry, K. (2007). *Rx for health care reform*. Nashville: Vanderbilt University Press.

The News Gram Newspaper (2012). Advertisement. Eagle Pass, Texas.

The Revolution Continues (2012). *Occupy Wall Street*. http://occupywallst.org/.

The Cochran Collaboration (2013). *The personalized risk communication for informed decision making about taking screening tests*. http://www.cochrane.org/features/personalised-risk-communication-informed-decision-making-about-taking-screening-tests.

Thomas, J. L., Cummings, J. L., and O'Donahue, W. T. (2002). *The entrepreneur in psychology*, The collected papers of Nicholas A. Cummings, Vol. II. Phoenix, AZ: Zeig, Tucker & Theisen, Inc.

Thomas, K. J. (2000). *American Banker*. September 1:13.

Thomma, S. (2009). *Distrust of government blunting Obama's pursuit of new programs*. McClatchy Newspapers. http://www.mcclatchydc.com/2009/07/24/72452/distrust-of-government-blunting.html#storylink=cpy.

Thompson, C. A. (2011). *Stakeholders in supply chain discuss shortages*. American Journal of Health System Pharmacy, 68, January 11. doi: 10.2146/news100088.

Thompson, D. (2012). *How the richest 400 people in America got so rich*. The Atlantic, July 12. http://finance.yahoo.com/news/richest-400-people-america-got-201519751.html.

Tuckfelt, S., Fink, J., Warren, M. P. (1997). *The psychotherapists' guide to managed care in the 21st century, surviving big brother and providing quality mental health services*. Northvale, New Jersey: Jason Aronson Inc.

Tulenko, K. (2012). *Healthcare's foreign invasion*. Salon, April 28. http://www.salon.com/2012/04/28/healthcares_foreign_invasion/.

U.S. Department of Homeland Security (2012). *State and major urban area fusion centers*. http://www.dhs.gov/files/programs/gc_1156877184684.shtm.

U.S. Department of Justice (2012). *Fact sheet: Justice Department Counter-Terrorism Efforts Since 9/11*. http://www.justice.gov/opa/pr/2008/September/08-nsd-807.html. www.healthcare.gov/law/timeline/full.html. Other resources include: IRS: Affordable Care Act Tax provisions, HealthReform.gov: The Affordable Care Act's New Patient's Bill of Rights; Health Care In Action. http://www.whitehouse.gov/healthreform/healthcare-overview. Key features of the Affordable Care Act, by year, www.healthcare.gov/law/timeline/full.html.

U. S. History (2012). *New York Stock Exchange*. http://www.u-s-history.com/pages/h1806.html http://en.wikipedia.org/wiki/List_of_federal_political_scandals_in_the_United_States.

Viscussi, W. K. (1992). *Fatal tradeoffs*, NY: Oxford University Press.

Viscusi, W. K. (2004) The Value of Life: Estimates with Risks by Occupation and Industry Economic Inquiry, 42,1, pages 29–48, January 2004.

Wallach, M. (2012). *The therapist as entrepreneur: An interview with Iris Lipner*. http://www.irislipnerlcsw.com/practice/entreprene ur.html.

Wall Street Journal (2009). *Government programs always exceed their spending estimates.* Review   and   Outlook.   http://online.wsj.com/article/ SB10001424052748703746604574461610985243066.html.

Weinberger, S. (2011). *Windfalls of war: Pentagon's no-bid contracts triple in 10 years of war.* iWatch News, The Center for Public Integrity. http://www.iwatchnews.org/national-security/windfalls-war

Weissert, C. S. and Weissert W. G. (2002). *Governing health, The politics of health policy,* 2nd Ed., Baltimore: The John Hopkins University Press.

Whaley, P. (2012). *You might think I'm crazy, but this is a really good time to start a solo practice, especially for primary care providers.* http://www.managemypractice.com/yes-you-can-and-should-start-a-solo-medical-practice-in-2013/.

White, C. R. (2007). *Health care meltdown, confronting the myths and fixing our failing system.* Quoted in the Foreward. Robert H. LeBow, author. Chambersburg, Pennsylvania: Alan C. Hood & Company, Inc.

White, L. J. 1991. *The S&L debacle: Public policy lessons for bank and thrift regulation.* Oxford University Press.

Withrow, C. (2012). *America's Affordable Health Care Act of 2009.* www.ehow.com/info_7796513_americas-health-care-act-2009.html. Other resources include: IRS: Affordable Care Act Tax provisions, HealthReform.gov: The Affordable Care Act's New Patient's Bill of Rights; Health Care In Action:. http://www.whitehouse.gov/healthreform/healthcare-overview.

Witkin, G. (1992). *Beware these health scams.* Reader's Digest, July, p. 142-146. Pleasanton, NY.

Wright, A. (2011). *Mental health labels and stigma: A survey of young people.* Psychiatry Weekly, 6, 23, on October 24, 2011. http://www.psychweekly.com/aspx/article/articledetail.aspx?articleid=1355.

About the Author

Ronald R. Hixson, PhD, has been a psychotherapist for over 30 years, first in the military and then in rural and border communities in South Texas. He has worked with a mental health hospital, started a group practice, and for the past six years has had a private practice. Dr. Hixson has been a columnist on practice management for the *Annals of Psychotherapy & Integrative Health* for nearly ten years. He is an active board member of two professional associations, American Pychotherapy Association and the American Mental Health Alliance, and has participated in workshops and seminars on the business side of therapy and other mental health issues. He has written two books, including his latest, *In the Practice of Health Care: The Search for Satisfaction*. Dr. Hixson's formal training includes three masters and one doctorate and he is currently enrolled in the doctorate of public health program at Capella University. He is an avid reader and enjoys writing. For leisure he works with his wife, Herlinda, on a small piece of heaven in Eagle Pass, Texas, which they share with two horses and a filly, their dog Lucky, many doves and birds, and even a few chickens.